Fundamentals of Glaucoma

A Guide for Ophthalmic Nurse Practitioners, Optometrists and Orthoptists

Other World Scientific Titles by the Author

Fundamentals of Intravitreal Injections: A Guide for Ophthalmic Nurse Practitioners and Allied Health Professionals
by Salman Waqar and Jonathan C. Park
ISBN: 978-981-3239-78-4
ISBN: 978-981-122-132-3 (pbk)

Intravitreal Injections: A Handbook for Ophthalmic Nurse Practitioners and Trainee Ophthalmologists
by Salman Waqar, Jonathan C. Park and Michael D. Cole
ISBN: 978-981-4571-45-6 (pbk)

Fundamentals of Glaucoma

A Guide for Ophthalmic Nurse Practitioners, Optometrists and Orthoptists

Edited by

Salman Waqar

FRCOphth
Consultant Ophthalmologist
Royal Eye Infirmary
Plymouth
United Kingdom

World Scientific

NEW JERSEY • LONDON • SINGAPORE • BEIJING • SHANGHAI • HONG KONG • TAIPEI • CHENNAI • TOKYO

Published by

World Scientific Publishing Co. Pte. Ltd.
5 Toh Tuck Link, Singapore 596224
USA office: 27 Warren Street, Suite 401-402, Hackensack, NJ 07601
UK office: 57 Shelton Street, Covent Garden, London WC2H 9HE

British Library Cataloguing-in-Publication Data
A catalogue record for this book is available from the British Library.

ISBN 978-981-121-644-2 (hardcover)
ISBN 978-981-121-746-3 (paperback)
ISBN 978-981-121-645-9 (ebook for institutions)
ISBN 978-981-121-646-6 (ebook for individuals)

For any available supplementary material, please visit
https://www.worldscientific.com/worldscibooks/10.1142/11718#t=suppl

CONTENTS

FOREWORD

Glaucoma care in the UK is changing. More than ever before are non-medical healthcare professionals such as nurses, orthoptists, and optometrists becoming involved in caring for patients — carrying out tests, interpreting results, and contributing to management decisions as part of a multi-disciplinary team. To work efficiently as part of a team, each professional needs to have a fundamental understanding of each other's role. This is particularly important when it comes to speaking with patients, some of whom will be anxious of having been diagnosed with a potentially sight-threatening disease. There are many excellent textbooks on glaucoma, but this book fills a gap for a simple and concise overview of clinical glaucoma care. It is written at a basic level that will not be intimidating to the novice, and the compact format will make it easy to use. It will be a useful resource for all of those who are beginning to enter this area and would like to build their knowledge.

Paul H Artes
PhD, MCOptom
Professor in Eye & Vision Sciences
Faculty of Health: Medicine, Dentistry, and Human Sciences
University of Plymouth

ACKNOWLEDGEMENTS

I am very grateful to all the contributors for taking time out of their busy clinical schedules to support a well-rounded, useful and relevant addition to the field of glaucoma. My sincere thanks also to Dr Rabia Salman for thoroughly proof-reading the text.

And, as always, our greatest appreciation for our patients who trust us to look after their vision and teach us something new at every step of our journeys.

LIST OF CONTRIBUTORS

Mr Imran Masood, Consultant Ophthalmologist, Birmingham and Midland Eye Centre, Birmingham, U.K.

Mr Michael Smith, Consultant Ophthalmologist, West of England Eye Unit, Exeter, U.K.

Mr Adam Booth, Consultant Ophthalmologist, Royal Eye Infirmary, Plymouth, U.K.

Mr Pierre Rautenbach, Consultant Ophthalmologist, Department of Ophthalmology, Royal Cornwall Hospitals NHS Trust, U.K.

Mrs Katie Smith, Specialist Optometrist, Bristol Eye Hospital, Bristol, U.K.

Mrs Pam Adams, Optometrist and LVA Clinic Supervisor, Department of Optometry and Vision Sciences, University of Plymouth, U.K.

Mr Abhijit A. Mohite, Glaucoma Fellow, Birmingham and Midland Eye Centre, Birmingham, U.K.

Mr Thomas Sherman, Specialist Registrar, South West Peninsula School of Ophthalmology, U.K.

Mr Neil Bowley, Specialist Registrar, South West Peninsula School of Ophthalmology, U.K.

Mr Andrew Swampillai, Specialist Registrar, South West Peninsula School of Ophthalmology, U.K.

ILLUSTRATIONS

Khadijah Azhar (www.khadijahazhar.com)

INTRODUCTION

Glaucoma is one of the commonest causes of visual impairment worldwide.

Ophthalmic Nurse Practitioners, Optometrists and Orthoptists are increasingly becoming invaluable team members for diagnosing, monitoring and treating glaucoma, particularly as the clinical demand increases.

This book has been written to assist our colleagues in such an endeavour, and it is hoped that it will provide concise but relevant information in a format that is easy to carry around and access. It is aimed primarily at nurse practitioners and allied health professionals, but we are confident that it will also be a useful reference for junior ophthalmic trainees learning about the condition.

We wish our readers all the best for their career as part of the glaucoma team!

1

ANATOMY

Pierre Rautenbach

In order to develop an understanding of the glaucomatous disease process and the treatment options available, it is imperative to have a good grasp of the basic anatomy and physiology of certain relevant parts of the eye.

The eye is an approximate sphere 2.5 cm in diameter (equivalent to an axial length of 25 mm) with a volume of 5 ml (it fills one-sixth of the orbit whose volume is 30 ml).

It is a highly specialised organ of photoreception. This is a process by which light energy from the environment produces changes in specialised nerve cells in the retina (rods and cones). These changes result in action potentials (the electrical voltage across a cell) that are subsequently relayed to the optic nerve and then to the brain where the information is processed and consciously appreciated as vision.

THE LAYERS OF THE EYE

The eye consists of 3 basic layers.

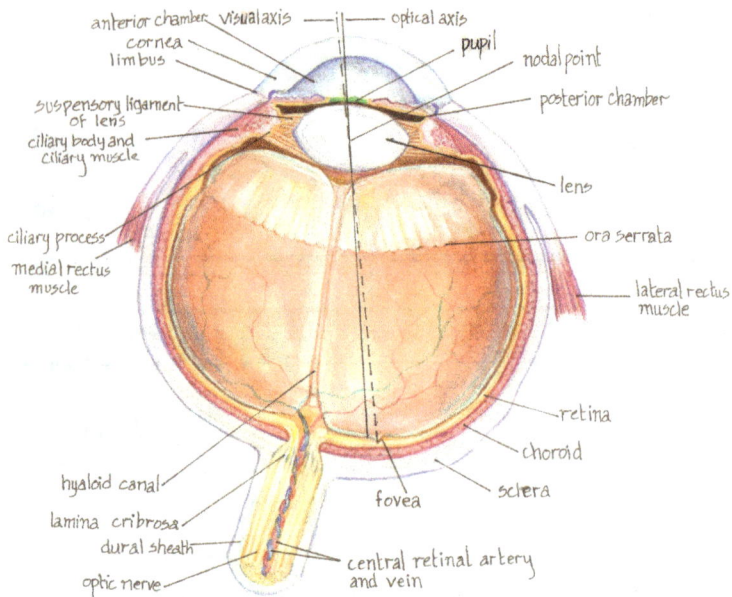

Fig. 1.1. The eye in cross section.

The Fibrous Corneoscleral Coat

It consists of the cornea and sclera.

- **The Cornea**

This is the anterior most transparent window of the eye. The cornea meets the sclera at the limbus, which is also where the conjunctiva ends. The conjunctiva covers the sclera but does not cover the cornea. The cornea is kept transparent by its avascularity and the innermost monolayer of cells (endothelium) which pumps fluid out of the corneal stroma. The cornea presents a tough barrier to trauma and infection and is responsible for about two-thirds of the eyes refractive power (the other one-third coming from the lens).

- **The Sclera**

This is an opaque white fibrous coat that also protects the eye and maintains its shape due to inherent structural integrity.

The Uvea (or Uveal Tract)

The middle vascular pigmented layer of the eye and consists of the iris, ciliary body and choroid.

- **The Iris**

This is a thin contractile circular disc, which is analogous to the diaphragm of a camera. The iris separates the anterior and posterior chambers, which are filled with aqueous humour and are in continuity through an opening, the pupil. The iris is attached by its root at the 'angle' (iridocorneal) of the anterior chamber where it merges with the ciliary body and trabecular meshwork. Aqueous humour drains mainly through the trabecular meshwork, which is visible using a mirror within a contact lens called a gonioscope.

- **The Ciliary Body**

This is approximately 6 mm in width and is responsible for the production of aqueous humour. It also contains muscles, which are attached to the zonular ligaments of the lens (changing its shape on contraction to focus or accommodate). It has two parts, the pars plicata and the pars plana. The pars plicata is the anterior part. It is 2 mm long (measured from the limbus) and contains about 70 ciliary processes which are the site of attachment for the aforementioned zonular ligaments. The pars plana is a posterior flat area which is 4 mm long. As the sclera and cornea are relatively rigid, excess production/reduced drainage of aqueous humour or injection of substances into the eye leads to raised intra-ocular pressure (normal is up to 21 mmHg). Intraocular pressure is high immediately after intravitreal injections (can be as high as 60 mmHg). Normalisation of the pressure usually occurs over 30 minutes after injection and is dependent on aqueous humour outflow through the trabecular meshwork.

• **The Choroid**

This highly pigmented and vascular posterior portion lies between the sclera and the retina and extends forward to the ciliary body. Its principal function is to nourish the outer layers of the retina and prevent unwanted light from reflecting back through the retina. It is composed of an outer layer of large calibre blood vessels, which divide into smaller diameter vessels and ultimately form the choriocapillaris (a network of capillaries). These drain into the vortex veins, which ultimately drain into the superior and inferior ophthalmic veins.

The Retina (Neural Layer)

This is where photoreception occurs and consists of two primary layers, the inner neurosensory retina and an outer layer called the retinal pigment epithelium. Anatomically the following regions are described:

• **The Macula** (Latin 'patch', same as macula lutea)

The area within the main vascular arcades and is 5–6 mm in diameter. Cone photoreceptors are mostly concentrated here for fine resolution (maximum density in the fovea).

• **The Fovea** (Latin: 'pit')

The central 1.5 mm diameter area of the macula. The foveola is the central 0.35 mm diameter area of the fovea.

- **The Optic Disc**

1.5 mm in diameter, it contains no normal retinal layers or photoreceptors (thus causing the blind spot) and is the area where nerve fibres of retinal ganglion cells pierce the sclera to enter the optic nerve. The central pale thinned area of the disc forms the cup, which becomes progressively enlarged through loss of ganglion cells in glaucoma. The cups vertical diameter is measured in relation to the disc diameter when monitoring patients with glaucoma (referred to as the cup to disc ratio).

- **The Peripheral Retina**

Rich in rod photoreceptors that provide acuity in low levels of illumination.

- **The Ora Serrata**

This is where the peripheral retina ends. It is approximately 7 mm from the limbus.

AQUEOUS HUMOUR

The aqueous humour is a clear fluid that fills the anterior segment of the eye. It has many vital functions. It provides nutrients and removes toxic waste products from all surrounding structures. It is clear, allowing light to pass unhindered and acts as a vehicle for important immunological cells and chemicals. It inflates the globe to maintain structural and functional integrity to all eye structures. The degree to which this is done can be measured as the intra ocular pressure (IOP). The IOP is therefore a delicate balance between the production and drainage of aqueous humour. This is normally regulated automatically by various mechanisms to produce an ideal IOP and good blood flow around the optic nerve head. In glaucoma there is an imbalance in this system. All glaucoma treatments are therefore designed to optimize and modify this pathway, specific to the patient being treated. Controlling the IOP is the only risk factor modification proven to prevent progression in glaucoma.

Aqueous Production

Aqueous fluid is actively produced by the ciliary body. Enzymes like Carbonic Anhydrase play an important role in this process. The fluid then circulates from the posterior to the anterior chamber through the pupil.

Aqueous Outflow

Drainage of the fluid takes place via two routes:

• Trabecular (Conventional) Route

This accounts for the majority (90%) of the outflow. The trabecular meshwork is a sieve-like structure in the angle between the peripheral iris and the cornea (also known as the iridocorneal angle). Aqueous passes through the trabecular meshwork into the Schlemm's Canal and then into the episcleral veins (Fig. 1.2). This route can be affected by changes in pressure in the eye and venous drainage around the eye. The higher the IOP the more the drainage, and the higher the episcleral venous pressure the less the drainage.

• Uveoscleral (Unconventional) Route

This accounts for the minority of the outflow (10%). Aqueous passes across the face of the ciliary body and iris into the suprachoroidal space and is thereafter drained by the venous system of the ciliary body, iris, choroid and sclera.

THE RETINA AND THE OPTIC NERVE HEAD

The retina's role in vision is to convert light energy as it falls on it into electrical energy. This is then transported from the eye along the optic nerves to the brain, so it can be appreciated.

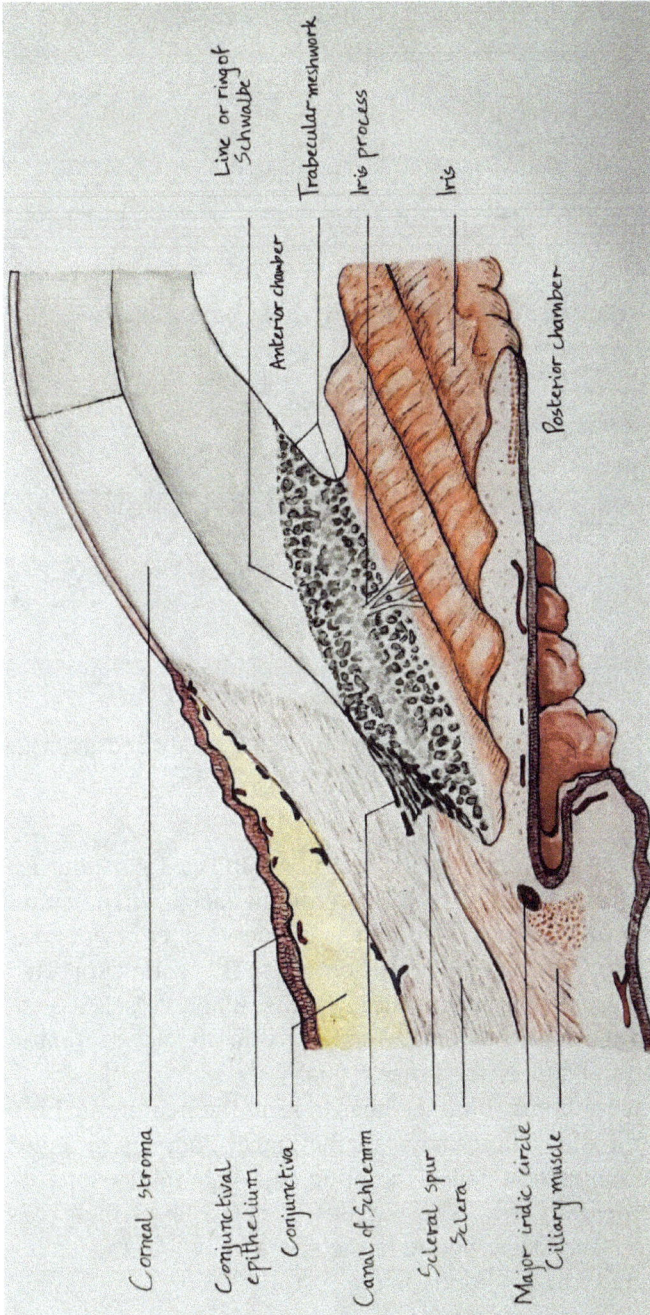

Fig. 1.2. Anatomy of the iridocorneal angle.

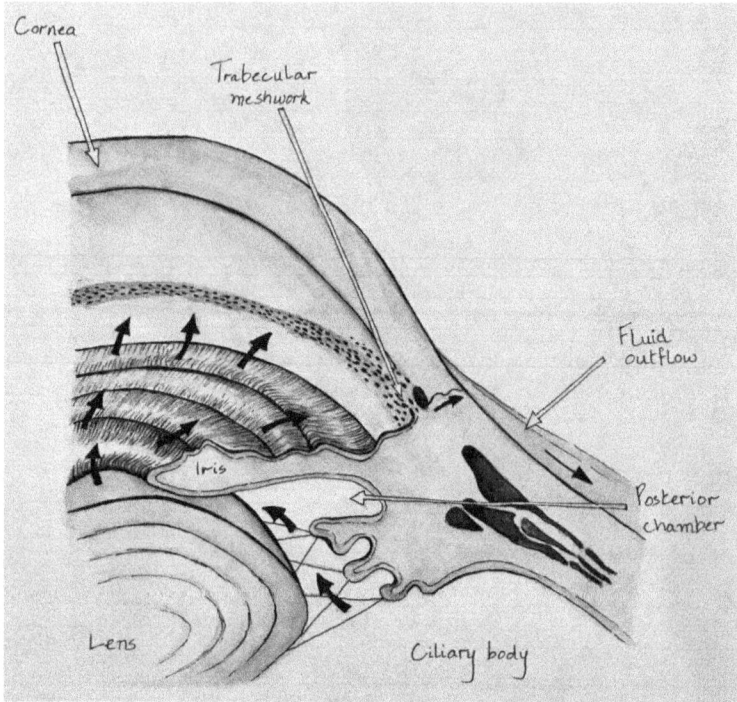

Fig. 1.3. Production of aqueous by the ciliary body and drainage through the Trabecular route (black arrows).

The various layers of the retina are shown in Fig. 1.4. About 1.2 million retinal ganglion cells are present in each eye. The innermost layer of the retina is known as the nerve fiber layer and is composed of axons of the ganglion cells. These are supported by glial cells without any myelin sheaths. Blood vessels associated with the central retinal artery and vein are also present in this layer and supply the inner retina.

The nerve fibres come together to form the neuroretinal rim of the optic disc before they exit the globe. They are arranged around a depression called the optic cup which does not contain any neural tissue. The bundles of nerve fibres then pass through a sieve-like structure in the sclera known as the lamina cribrosa and form the optic nerve.

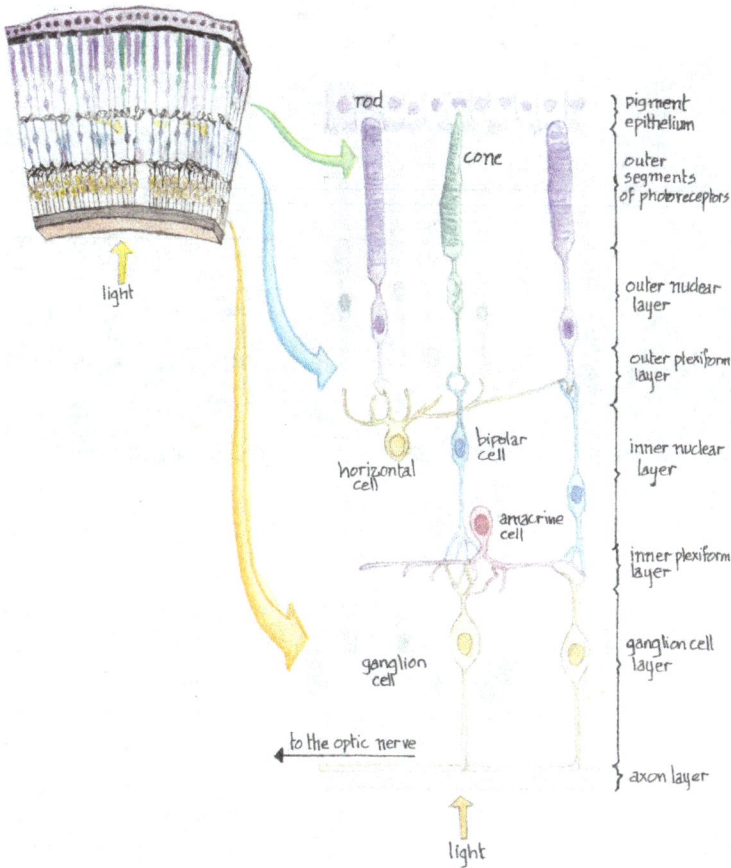

Fig. 1.4. The retina in cross section (note the Nerve Fibre Layer has been labelled as the Axon Layer).

Clinically, the neuroretinal rim is seen as an area between the edge of the cup and the margin of the disc. It is pink in colour and represents the nerve fibre layer changing course by ninety degrees to enter the sclera (Fig. 1.5).

The central retinal artery and vein enter and exit the disc centrally and then course nasally before diving into Superior, Inferior, Nasal and Temporal branches.

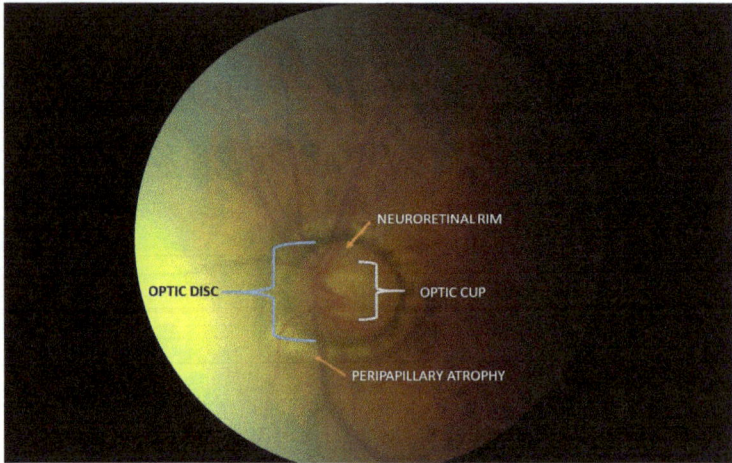

Fig. 1.5. Optic disc.

The cup to disc ratio (CDR) describes the diameter of the cup compared to the disc. It is expressed as a fraction; e.g. 0.5 means 50% of the diameter of the disc is occupied by neuroretinal rim. This is an important clinical sign as an increase in this raises the suspicion of glaucoma. Traditionally, a ratio of above 0.5 is regarded as suspicious of glaucoma. It is however important to note that the size of the scleral canal is often proportional to the size of the globe. In myopia (short sightedness) the globe and the scleral canal tend to be larger, but the amount of ganglion cells remains constant. Retinal nerve fibres therefore pass out of the eye through a more generous space at the periphery of the disc, which can lead to a physiologically increased CDR ratio. Similarly, hypermetropes (long sightedness) with smaller eyes can give the impression of a reduced CDR.

A temporal crescent of chorio-retinal atrophy around the optic disc can occur in up to eighty percent of the normal population and is common in high myopia. However, this phenomenon is more common, and the area tends to be larger, in glaucoma.

Detailed understanding of the optic nerve heads blood supply is not required here, but it is important to have some knowledge since interruption to it can result in damage to the optic nerve. The main source of blood supply is from the short posterior ciliary arteries, which in turn are branches of the ophthalmic artery. However, the nerve fibre layer visible within the eye is supplied by the retinal circulation. The flow of blood around the nerve is automatically regulated to ensure normal fluctuations in IOP, blood pressure and cerebrospinal fluid pressure have a minimal effect on blood flow. If this regulation is interrupted or the changes are too extreme to cope with, blood supply to the optic nerve head can be compromised and ischemic irreversible damage to the nerve fibres could occur. This often results in disc pallour, and the astute clinician must be able to differentiate this from glaucomatous changes, as further investigations and treatment will vary according to the underlying condition.

THE LENS

The lens is a highly organised system of specialised cells within a transparent capsule. Situated in the anterior segment of the eye it provides a third of the refractive power of the eye. Zonules from the ciliary body hold the lens in place.

A cataract (Latin for 'waterfall') is regarded as a visually significant opaqueness of the lens for which age is the most common risk factor. Development of a cataract can lead to narrowing of the iridocorneal angle, which, in turn, can cause both acute or chronic angle closure glaucoma.

2

DEFINITION AND CLASSIFICATION

Neil Bowley

Glaucoma has been known since antiquity, and yet a full understanding of the pathophysiological mechanisms is not known today; it is probable that an interplay of environmental and genetic factors results in the clinical presentation of glaucoma.

Glaucoma is a syndrome in which progressive damage occurs to the ganglion cells which form the optic nerve, therefore producing a corresponding visual field defect. The etiology of this damage is multifactorial. A combination of raised intraocular pressure, ischaemic injury, autoimmune dysregulation, trans-cribriform plate pressure differential and excitotoxicity have been postulated as contributory factors.

Most commonly, raised pressure within the eye is a key factor in developing glaucoma; however, elevated intraocular pressure and glaucoma are **not** synonyms. This misconception is common both with patients and non-ophthalmic medical professionals.

It is possible to have raised intraocular pressure and no glaucomatous nerve damage; similarly, it is possible to have a measured intraocular pressure within the 'normal' range and still have a progressive nerve damage.

The intraocular pressure is maintained by the secretion of the aqueous and its drainage as shown in Equation 1.

$$IOP = \left[\frac{(Aqueous\,formation - uveoscleral\,outflow)}{trabecular\,meshwork\,outflow + episcleral\,venous\,pressure} \right]$$

Equation 1. Intraocular pressure (IOP) calculation

A 'normal' intraocular pressure is between 10 and 21 mmHg, which encompasses 95% of the normal population.

A gross simplification of the flow of aqueous within the eye is shown in Fig. 2.1. The aqueous is produced by the ciliary body (shown in pink) at a rate of approximately 2.5 µl per minute (normal AC volume is approximately 170 µl). The aqueous passes between the posterior surface of the iris and the anterior lens, then on through the pupil into the anterior chamber of the eye. The aqueous is primarily returned to the episcleral veins by filtration through the trabecular meshwork, which is located at the interface of the anterior iris and the cornea, known as 'the angle'. The 'uveo-scleral' outflow pathway, which does not rely on the trabecular meshwork, plays a smaller role in the recycling of aqueous. The aqueous is absorbed by the iris and the sclera directly and is returned passively to the blood.

The classification and correct identification of the specific type of glaucoma the patient has is important because it will alter how the patient's condition is managed and the likely clinical course. The specific diagnosis can be made clinically with examination and testing as discussed in the following chapters.

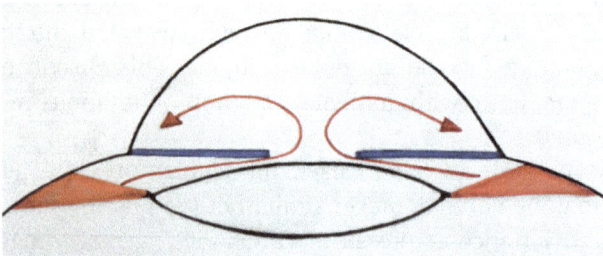

Fig. 2.1. Normal movement of aqueous within the eye.

Currently; medical, LASER, and surgical therapies available to us rely on manipulation of the secretion, reabsorption and movement of the aqueous humour within, and out of the eye. Therefore, the classification of glaucomatous disease will focus on this anatomical and etiological mechanism. Two large sub-classifications of glaucoma are therefore possible; if the flow of aqueous present within the eye under study is unimpeded from ciliary body to the iridocorneal angle, the glaucoma is said to be 'open angle'; if this passage of aqueous is structurally impeded, the glaucoma is defined as 'closed angle'.

OCULAR HYPERTENSION

Ocular hypertension is a condition where the measured intraocular pressure is higher than 24 mmHg, but no glaucomatous visual field loss or optic nerve damage has occurred. In the landmark Ocular Hypertension Study (OHTS) there was shown to be a 5-year risk of conversion to glaucoma in approximately 9.5% of patients. Factors which increase the risk of conversion to glaucoma (and therefore increase probability of starting treatment) include:

• Higher pressure at presentation.
• Older age at presentation.
• Thinner corneas.
• Increased cup/disc ratio.
• Afro-Caribbean heritage.
• Males are more likely to convert to glaucoma than females.

CLOSED ANGLE GLAUCOMA

If the flow of aqueous is impeded, the resulting glaucoma is said to be 'closed angle' as the trabecular meshwork is obstructed (Fig. 2.2). This is the underlying pathological mechanism in primary angle closure, phacomorphic glaucoma and inflammatory processes which result in 360° posterior

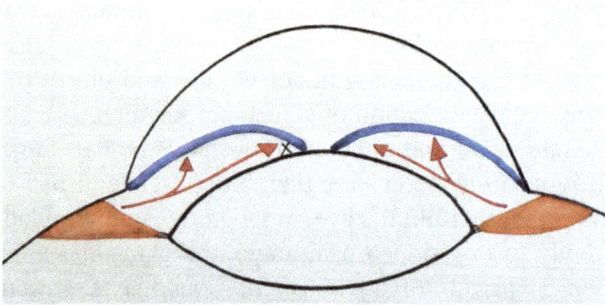

Fig. 2.2. Restriction of aqueous flow.

synechiae (adhesions of the iris at the pupillary margin and the anterior lens).

Primary Angle Closure

Primary angle closure glaucoma is due to the iridocorneal angle (and therefore trabecular meshwork) being occluded by the iris. Primary angle closure is more common in hyperopic persons, because the iridocorneal angle is more acute at baseline.

The clinical presentation of the patient with primary angle closure glaucoma is either acute with severe symptoms or chronic, which may be asymptomatic.

The chief symptom of acute primary angle closure is an extremely painful red eye, which is due to raised pressure within the eye (usually in the range of 50–100 mmHg). Due to the severity of the symptoms, patients often present to the A&E Department and initially diagnoses of subarachnoid haemorrhage or cluster headache are often considered.

Characteristic clinical signs are a deeply injected eye and opaque cornea. The cornea is often oedematous due to the corneal endothelial pumps being overwhelmed by the significant hydrostatic pressure from the anterior chamber. The iris is fixed and usually mid-dilated due to a combination of ischemia and inflammatory reaction. There is an inflammatory component due to the ischaemic damage to the iris causing breakdown of the blood-aqueous barrier. This inflammation can cause adhesions between the iris and lens (posterior synechiae) or between the iris and cornea (peripheral anterior synechiae).

Breaking this attack medically is the first stage in management, which should be followed by laser iridotomy and/or surgical lens extraction and intraocular lens insertion, which will be covered in more detail in later chapters.

There may be chronic angle closure where the pressure within the eye has been raised for many months or years due to partial occlusion of the trabeculum. This is usually asymptomatic. Definitive management is lens extraction to make more space within the anterior chamber.

It is possible to have narrow iridocorneal angles without raised pressure and without signs of glaucoma. The risk of developing high pressure with this anatomical configuration is significant, and prophylactic laser peripheral iridotomies are often performed if there is greater than 180° of Shaeffer Grade 1 or 0 on the gonioscopy.

In plateau iris syndrome, anteriorly rotated ciliary body processes can push the peripheral iris forward thereby causing narrowing of the iridocorneal angle.

Phacomorphic Angle Closure Glaucoma

This situation can present acutely with an 'angle closure' type event (described above) or more insidiously. As one ages, the lens of the eye continues to grow and thicken. This reduces the space within the anterior chamber of the eye and can cause bowing forward of the iris and occlusion of the trabeculum (Fig. 2.2).

Treatment is focused on removing the cataractous lens once the intraocular pressure has been normalized medically. A peripheral iridotomy may be a temporizing measure, whilst waiting for surgery.

Secondary Angle Closure

Secondary angle closure may be generated by any swelling of the posterior chamber of the eye, for example; iris/ciliary body/choroidal tumours, choroidal effusions secondary to chorio-retinal inflammation/scleritis or choroidal haemorrhage. Treatment is directed towards removing the provoking stimulus if possible.

It can also be caused by intraocular inflammation, whereby adhesions between the peripheral iris and the cornea (known as peripheral anterior synechiae) can contract and close the iridocorneal angle. This mechanism is also seen with fibro-vascular sheets that can develop within the iridocorneal angle in neovascular glaucoma and close the angle.

The use of the anti-epileptic medication, Topiramate, can cause bilateral ciliary body oedema, thereby causing angle closure. Treatment is directed towards cessation of Topiramate and medical control of the intraocular pressure until the oedema resolves.

OPEN ANGLE GLAUCOMA

Primary Open Angle Glaucoma (POAG)

Primary open angle glaucoma is the most frequently diagnosed of the glaucoma syndromes. Patients are usually asymptomatic until the later stages of their disease, unless a paracentral scotoma is present. In the absence of other neurological reasons for the visual impairment, the diagnosis is made by a triad of clinical signs:

- Open angles gonioscopically.
- Glaucomatous damage to the optic nerve with corresponding field defect.
- Raised intraocular pressure (> 21 mmHg).

The clinical signs and resulting visual field defects are discussed in more detail in later chapters.

Treatment is aimed at reducing the intraocular pressure either medically (drops), by laser (SLT/ALT), or surgically (e.g. trabeculectomy or aqueous shunt device). Reducing the IOP has been shown to reduce progression of glaucomatous field defects.

Prognosis is important to discuss with the patient when first diagnosing the condition and may be the source of concerns at future visits. Most POAG patients will not go blind within their lifetime due to glaucoma if the condition is optimally managed.

Normal Tension Glaucoma (NTG)

Normal tension glaucoma is a variant of POAG where glaucomatous damage to the optic nerve occurs at 'normal' pressures. The central corneal thickness must be accounted for, which, if significantly below 520 μm, can mean that the Goldmann pressure measurement is significantly underestimated. Also consider that if the patient is on a systemic beta blocker there will be some IOP lowering effect of this medication, thereby taking a previously diagnosed NTG patient into a pressure range in keeping with POAG. Visual field defects close to fixation are more common in this cohort of patients.

The differential diagnosis of glaucoma must be considered before a final diagnosis of NTG is made, and the practitioner must be confident that the probability of alternative etiologies is as low as possible, by careful history taking and thorough clinical examination.

Differential diagnosis:

- Progressive structural neurological disease — can be effectively ruled out with MRI brain.
- Previous anterior ischaemic optic neuropathy.
- Previous neurological insult, such as severe head trauma or septicemic shock, which results in either compressive or ischaemic optic nerve damage.
- Previously raised IOP e.g. due to acute anterior uveitis, or steroid use (peri-ocularly or systemically at high dose).

Pressure lowering is of benefit for some patients, but significant progression of visual field loss can still occur with pressures in the mid-teens. If a 30% reduction in IOP from the baseline is achieved, 80% of patients achieve stability and no progression of their visual field defects.

Secondary Open Angle Glaucoma

This may be classified based on the site of the anatomical abnormality causing raised intraocular pressure as follows:

• **Trabecular Secondary Open Angle Glaucoma**

This is caused by dysfunction of the trabeculum. The trabecular meshwork may be obstructed by deposited material such as pseudoexfoliation, pigment from pigment dispersion or lens protein from phacolytic glaucoma.

Pseudoexfoliation glaucoma is an important diagnosis to make for both prognostic reasons and for surgical planning. The signs and symptoms are discussed in the clinical examination chapter. A fine filamentous deposit is lain down on the internal structures of the eye. This clogs the trabecular meshwork and weakens the zonular fibres.

The trabeculum can become inflamed especially in herpetic disease (*Herpes zoster*) or in Posner-Schlossman syndrome. These conditions usually respond well to administration of topical steroids.

The trabeculum can become dysfunctional due to the administration of steroids, either topically or systemically. This causes a secondary pressure increase and may result in glaucomatous nerve damage if left untreated. Patients with POAG appear to be more sensitive to developing steroid-response pressure rises.

• **Post-trabecular Secondary Open Angle Glaucoma**

Increased episcleral venous pressure causes increased intraocular pressure. If the pressure is too high for too long, ganglion cell damage can occur. Examples of diseases causing raised episcleral venous pressure are: carotid-cavernous fistula, dysthyroid orbitopathy and Sturge-Weber Syndrome. If the underlying causative pathology can be treated, the IOP can normalize, and glaucomatous field damage progression can be halted.

3

EXAMINATION TECHNIQUES

Neil Bowley

Good clinical examination is critical for the effective management of patients with glaucoma. The important question to ask is: 'what information do I require and what is the most reliable way of getting it?'

Patients and clinicians have different ideas regarding what is an effective clinical encounter in a glaucoma clinic. The intention of this chapter is to discuss the 'mechanics' of clinical examination. The practitioner can *and must* modify their practice according to the patient who is in front of them.

This chapter is arranged according to a patient's imagined journey through an eye clinic at the Royal Eye Infirmary, Derriford Hospital. Each section includes:

- How examinations are usually performed.
- How to interpret the result.
- Key considerations which should be taken into account.

No single aspect of the examination can be taken in isolation. The *'gestalt'* needs to be the preferred mode of practice, *i.e.* the whole examination put together is greater than the sum of the parts. This must then be formulated into a management plan, tailored to the needs of the patient.

VISUAL ACUITY

This test is limited by the responses given by the patient; therefore, patients must be pressed to perform to their limit. If this is not done the visual acuity is an unreliable measure of progression.

- Patients should be tested with the most up-to-date refractive correction for distance, usually at 6 metres using an ETDRS or Snellen chart.
- A decrease may be due to media opacity (cornea, lens, posterior capsular opacification *etc.*), out of date prescription, ocular surface disorders (dry eye, surface disruption), and progression of central scotoma.
- If you did not perform this yourself and the result is rather unexpected, ask the patient if they were wearing their correct spectacles and if they were comfortable in doing the test. Consider repeating the test yourself.

PERMIETRY AND IMAGING

Automated testing of peripheral visual fields is a key aspect of the examination in a glaucoma clinic.

OCT imaging of the optic nerve is a relatively new technique. It involves using light-based scanning of the retina surrounding the optic nerve to assess the thickness of the nerve fibres heading towards the optic nerve, since these are the components damaged in glaucoma.

Care needs to be taken when interpreting the scans because it is based on a normative database which varies according to the manufacturer of the scanning machine. This database may not be representative of the population you are treating in terms of ethnicity or age. These investigations will be covered in more detail in the next chapter.

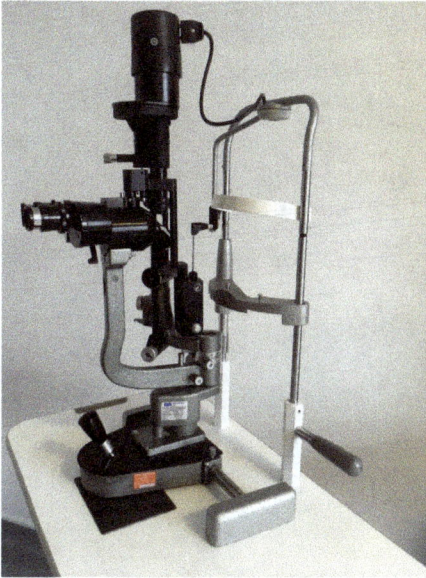

Fig. 3.1. Slit lamp.

SLIT LAMP

The slit lamp (Fig. 3.1) is a key piece of equipment which allows, with practice, quick and easy assessment of the patient's clinical status.

Systematic clinical examination is necessary, moving anterior to posterior.

Some common clinical findings are as follows:

Lids

Take care to inspect the lashes (and their position), lid margin and meibomian orifices.

Periocular pigmentation, lash lengthening and orbital fat atrophy are common side effects of long-term prostaglandin analogue use. Blepharitis, meibomian gland dysfunction and lid margin inflammation are a common side effect of many topical

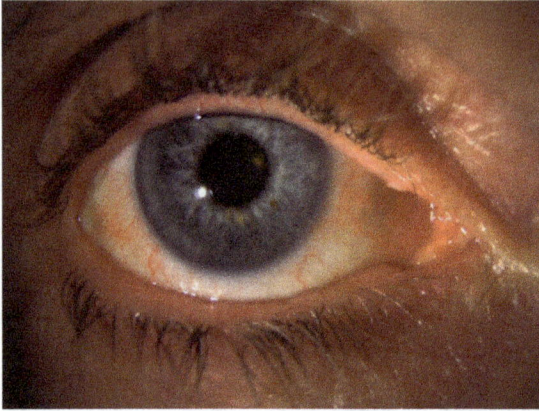

Fig. 3.2. Patient on long term prostaglandin analogue showing lash lengthening, hyperaemia of conjunctiva, and meibomian gland dysfunction.

anti-glaucoma medications (Fig. 3.2). These can be especially troublesome symptoms for the patients who suffer chronic irritation of the ocular surface. They can be alleviated (in part) by considering switching to a preservative free preparation or changing the medication. Non-pharmacological methods of pressure lowering (including Selective Laser Trabeculoplasty) may be undertaken to reduce the burden of drops.

Conjunctiva

Take care to inspect the superior limbus and the fornices.

Hyperaemia of the conjunctiva is a common side effect of anti-glaucoma medications. In particular the alpha agonist brimonidine is renowned for this. Look under the superior lid for a trabeculectomy bleb or filtration device. If there has been glaucoma surgery, ensure the conjunctiva is of a satisfactory thickness and there is no leak of aqueous by adding a drop of fluorescein to the conjunctival sac and looking for dilution of the fluorescein (Seidel's test). If there is a leak of aqueous this will require surgical attention due to the risk of intraocular infection.

Cornea

Look at the cornea with a light beam both wide and as thin as is possible to assess firstly the global health of the cornea and the location of any clinical features you wish to identify or inspect more closely. Apply fluorescein to the conjunctival sac. Wait a few seconds before continuing the examination to allow staining to occur.

Epithelial disruption is common and is sometimes due to drop therapy (see above for switching to Preservative Free preparations).

Look at the endothelium:

- *A brownish pigment on the endothelium may occur in pigment dispersion glaucoma.*
- *Pale white/cream deposits are seen in pseudoexfoliation.*
- *Keratic precipitates can be a result of intraocular inflammation.*

Anterior Chamber (Also see note on gonioscopy)

Note the central depth of the anterior chamber; this will become more obvious with experience. Take care to look for any cells which may indicate intraocular inflammation. This is achieved by:

- Making the room as dark as possible.
- Setting the beam on the slit lamp to maximum brightness and 1 × 1 mm in size.
- Setting the magnification to at least × 16.
- Setting the slit beam to enter the eye at approximately 45°.
- Bringing the cornea into focus then moving the slit lamp forwards to focus on the anterior chamber of the eye. Once the iris is in focus move the slit lamp back towards you a small amount using the joystick.
- Looking for cells that appear like dust in a shaft of light.

If intraocular inflammation is present, this may be the cause of the patient's glaucoma and if apparent, may need treating to control the pressure.

Iris

Look for abnormality of pupil size, shape or reaction. Take care to look for evidence of previous laser or surgery as this may be subtle, e.g. peripheral iridotomy (usually, but not exclusively between 10 and 2 o-clock). Iris transillumination is achieved by shining a pupil- sized bright co-axial slit beam through the pupil and looking at the light that shines back through the iris (retro-illumination).

If there is a peripheral iridotomy present, check by transillumination: Is the PI patent? Is it peripheral enough? Is it large enough?

Albinism, pseudoexfoliation syndrome and pigment dispersion syndrome can result in iris transillumination (radial and peripheral in pigment dispersion syndrome, radial and more central in pseudoexfoliation syndrome) (Fig. 3.3).

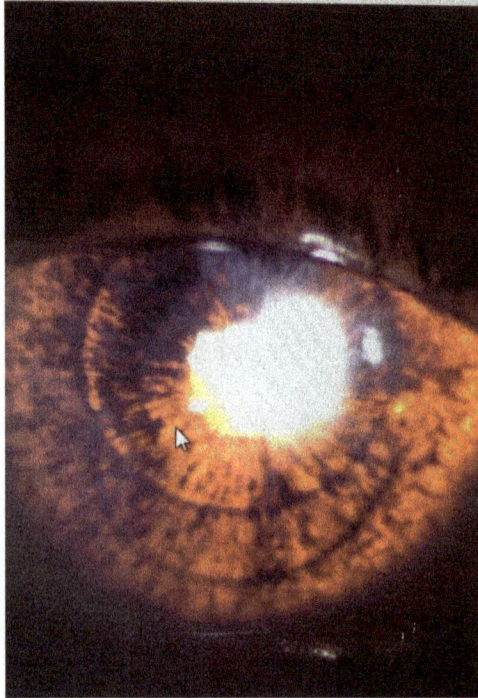

Fig. 3.3.   Iris transillumination.

Lens

It is best inspected with a dilated pupil in order to properly assess lenticular opacities. Using a narrow beam with the slit lamp arm set to 45° will give a 'cross sectional' view through the lens (Fig. 3.4). Retro-illumination gives the best view of posterior subcapsular cataracts.

Does the patient have a cataract? There is a significant demographic overlap due to the age of patients who have glaucoma and cataract. Sometimes the patient's symptoms can be attributed primarily to cataract.

Narrow angles or previous angle closure glaucoma can be due to the presence of a cataractous lens causing the iris to bow forwards, shallowing the anterior chamber.

Posterior segment

A good view of the posterior segment takes practice in addition to clear media. If the view is not clear, this may be indicative

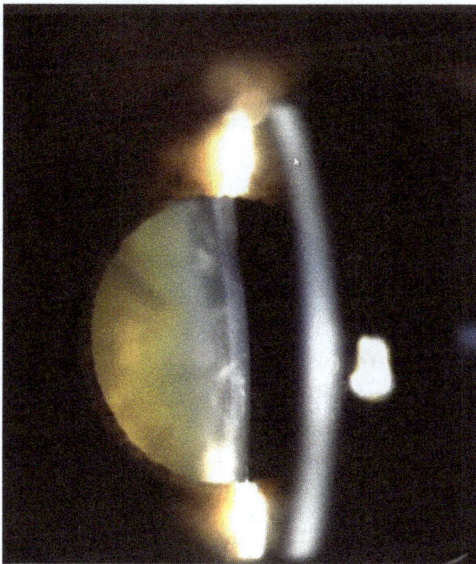

Fig. 3.4. Dense cortical and nuclear sclerotic cataract in glaucoma patient complaining of decreased vision.

of a second pathology, other than glaucoma, which is affecting the patient's vision. Most practitioners use a 90D or 78D Volk lens, which produces an inverted mirror image of the fundus (upside down and back to front), so what appears to you at the top of the view is the inferior retina.

Start by looking at the optic nerve head, then progress onto inspecting the macula to assess the general health of the patient's eye.

Inspection of the optic nerve requires a systematic approach. Things to look for are:

- Vertical size; can be measured with the slit lamp beam. Ensure you note which posterior segment lens (60D/78D/90D) you are using because they have different magnifications. A 60D lens has a magnification factor of 1 which means the disc size is what you have measured. 78D and 90D lenses minimise the image; therefore the measured value has to be multiplied by 1.1 and 1.3, respectively, to get the true optic nerve head size. This is important for contextualising the cup/disc ratio which is observed.
- Insertion; sometimes the optic nerve is not inserted straight into the sclera and results in a tilted appearance to the optic nerve head. This makes interpretation of the disc clinically much more difficult. This is more common in myopic patients.
- Cup to disc (C/D) ratio; the optic nerve cup is the central depression within the optic nerve head and it often appears more yellow/white in colour. The C/D ratio is calculated by measuring the vertical size of both the cup and the disc using a slit-lamp beam and then performing the mathematical division. In reality though, this is often a subjective judgement on the clinician's part rather than an objective calculation. In glaucomatous optic nerve damage, this ratio is increased with progressive enlargement of the optic nerve cup.

Normally the thickness of the nerve fibres decreases according to the 'ISNT' mnemonic — from thickest to thinnest: Inferiorly, Superiorly, Nasally, Temporally.

The cup/disc ratio needs to be taken in context of the size of the optic nerve. If the disc is small, the cup is correspondingly smaller because the same number of retinal nerve fibres are passing through a smaller area of the disc. Similarly, if the disc is large, a greater cup/disc ratio is acceptable.

- Peri-papillary atrophy; this is due to defects within the retinal pigment epithelium (the outermost layer of the retina) around the optic nerve. This may be indicative of glaucomatous damage, but also can be present in high myopia.
- Disc margin haemorrhages; more common is normal tension glaucoma and indicative of nerve fibre layer damage.
- Blood vessels emerging from disc; 'baring of blood vessels' is present when the optic disc cup is enlarged. Blood vessels travelling horizontally from the central vasculature no longer travel along the rim of the cup. 'Bayonetting' of blood vessels is where the vessels appear to 'double back' on their original direction.

Ensure you take time to inspect the macula because, as with cataract, there is a significant demographic overlap between the populations of patients suffering with glaucoma and age-related macular degeneration, which can cause a decrease in vision and the presence of central scotoma.

Clear documentation of your findings is vital, as changes in the appearance of the optic nerve can indicate glaucomatous progression, which would require modification of the treatment.

INTRAOCULAR PRESSURE MEASUREMENT

Goldmann Applanation Tonometry

There are a variety of pressure measuring techniques, all of which have their place; however the gold-standard is Goldmann applanation tonometry.

Intraocular pressure varies diurnally and with blood pressure, respiration and many other factors. Ideally glaucoma should not be managed solely on the basis of a single pressure measurement, sometimes taken 6–9 months after the last measurement. In reality however, logistical pressures may mean that this is the methodology commonly used.

Goldmann tonometry relies upon the mechanical principle that the tension of the tonometer arm required to flatten a specific area of the cornea is proportional to the intraocular pressure.

Procedure:

- A mixture of fluorescein and local anaesthetic is instilled (proxymetacaine stings less than lignocaine).
- Select cobalt blue light filter.
- The tonometer is brought into position (as in Fig. 3.5).
- The tonometer head is lightly applied to the central cornea.
- Two green mires appear in the view (Fig. 3.5). The thickness of the mires is important. If the mires are too thick (due to too much fluorescein) the pressure will be overestimated.
- When the mires are equal in size the central cornea is in contact with the tonometer.
- The pressure on the tonometer is adjusted so that the internal surfaces of the mires just meet. This is the intraocular pressure.

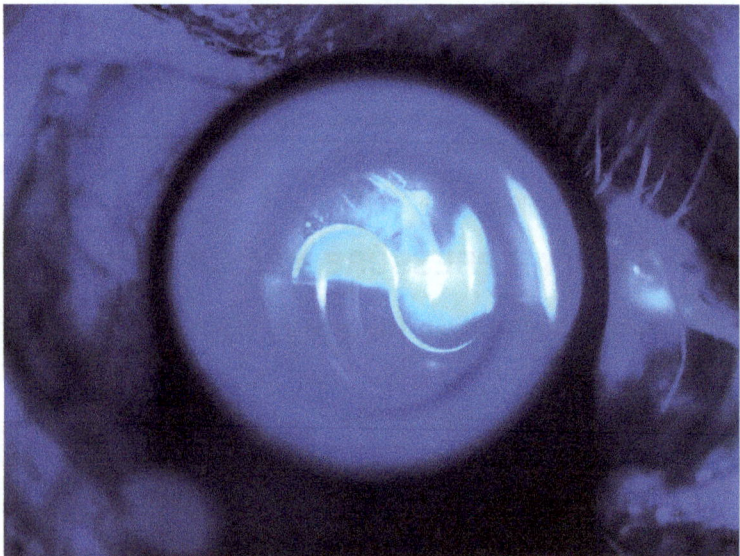

Fig. 3.5. Goldmann tonometry mires.

If your patient is not able to sit at the slit lamp, or GAT is difficult for other reasons, there are a variety of alternative methods to use to measure the pressure. Be sure to document the examination technique used, so that subsequent clinical examinations are comparable.

Tono-pen®

The Tono-pen is useful in immobile patients as it works at any angle. It is also useful in scarred corneas and is able to measure the intraocular pressure through bandage contact lenses.

Procedure:

- Ensure that the Tono-pen is working and is calibrated before you start.
- Instil anaesthetic drops.
- The instrument tip is covered with a sterile sheath (blue 'Ocu-Film' in Fig. 3.6).
- The instrument tip is then repeatedly applied gently to the central cornea until it gives a beep. It is important to measure

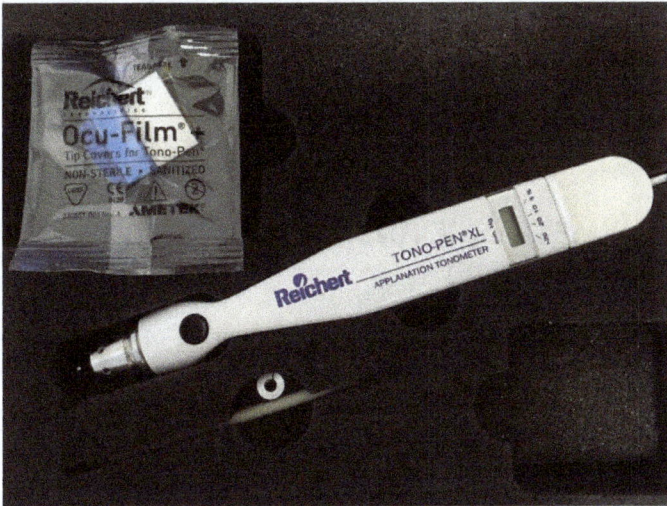

Fig. 3.6. Tono-pen.

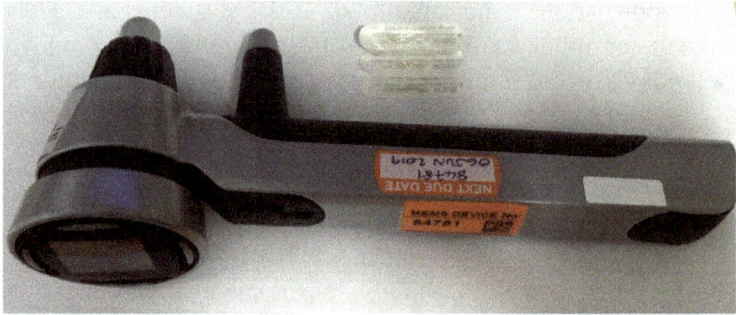

Fig. 3.7. iCare tonometer and probes.

the centre of the cornea because the cornea becomes thicker towards the limbus.

• The pressure will be displayed on the screen.

icare®

The iCare tonometer works by rebounding a small probe from the centre of the cornea. It is quick, easy, repeatable, and no drops required, making it extremely useful in children. It displays self-explanatory instructions on the screen when switched on. Depending on the model that your department has, the probe must either be parallel to the floor (all models) or may be used so that the probe is perpendicular to the floor (only some models). Taking measurements is not possible when the tonometer is angled.

PACHYMETRY (CORNEAL THICKNESS MEASUREMENT)

The thickness of the cornea is a vital piece of the jigsaw of patient management. This is because it influences the likelihood of glaucomatous progression and the correction factor, which has to be taken into account when measuring the intraocular pressure.

If a cornea is very thick, the pressure measured on applanation tonometry will be higher than is actually the case and vice

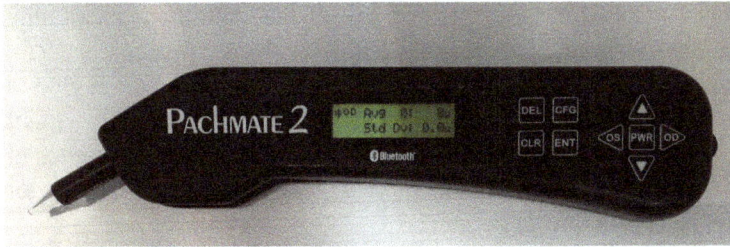

Fig. 3.8. Pachmate pachymeter.

versa. This is because the calculations on which tonometry is based take into consideration the thickness of the cornea.

Thicker cornea = More pressure required to deform during pressure measurement = Falsely raised IOP measurement

The central corneal thickness can be measured in a variety of ways. Optically an anterior segment Optical Coherence Tomography or Pentacam® scan can be taken and the thickness measured. There are also widely available hand-held ultra-sound pachymeters such as the Pachmate® (Fig. 3.8). These are quick and easy to use and give reliable results.

For handheld pachymetry:

- Tell the patient what to expect (i.e. that the probe will get close, and that it will not be painful, and to keep fixing on a distant point).
- Instil a drop of local anaesthetic.
- Get the patient to rest their head against the headrest of the seat.
- Lightly applanate the tip of the probe perpendicular to the central cornea. It is good practice to support the hand you use to hold the pachymeter against the patient's forehead (in case of sudden movement).
- The device takes 25 measurements within a couple of seconds and gives the average and standard deviation.

The average central corneal thickness in the healthy adult population is approximately 550 μm. Tables with correction factors for Goldmann Tonometer readings exist, but their exact utility in day to day practice remains debatable. Nonetheless, it is useful for the clinician to be aware of the corneal thickness as it gives a guide to the accuracy of the readings and can guide subsequent setting of target intraocular pressures. In addition, the presence of thin corneas has been confirmed to be an independent risk factor for glaucoma progression.

GONIOSCOPY

All new referrals to the glaucoma clinic should have gonioscopy performed if possible, as should patients with documented narrow angles or that have undergone laser peripheral iridotomy.

Gonioscopy takes practice to do and interpret properly. There are a variety of gonioscopy lenses, however the most common (and easiest to learn) lens type is the Goldmann Goniolens (Fig. 3.9).

Procedure:

- Tell the patient what you are going to do and what to expect because good patient cooperation is essential. Always dim room lights to allow for assessment of the iridocorneal angle with the pupil to be as dilated as possible.
- Put anaesthetic into the eye to be examined (e.g. Proxymetacaine 0.5%).
- Ask the patient to place their chin on the rest and forehead against the strap of the slit lamp and look where you tell them.
- Put a small amount of coupling agent (Carbomer 0.2%) onto the curved surface of the goniolens. Tell the patient this may run down their cheek during the examination and it is nothing to worry about.
- Ask patient to look up.
- Apply lens to eye (in one swift motion), then ask the patient to look straight ahead ensuring cornea is centred in the lens.
- It is most important is not to press too hard on the eye with the goniolens as this will distort the anatomy.
- Ask the patient to take a breath in and out (it is not uncommon for patients to hold their breath).

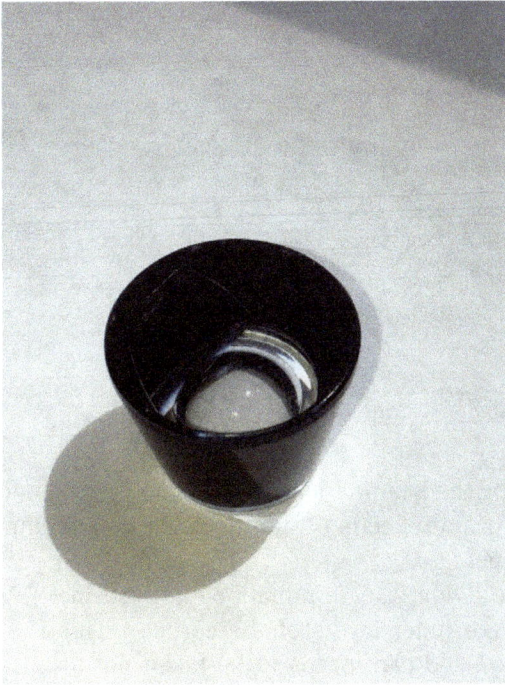

Fig. 3.9. Goldmann 1 mirror goniolens.

- Look into the lens at the mirror(s) and you are looking at the opposite angle, so if you are looking at the mirror when it is superior, you are, of course, looking at the inferior angle.

Interpretation:
The key sign to be able to elicit from gonioscopy is the most posterior visible ocular anatomical landmark, because this has implications as to the diagnosis and treatment of the patient. This is shown in Fig. 3.10 with the stick-man drawing showing the perspective achieved with the goniolens.

From anterior to posterior the angle structures in order are:

- *Corneal Wedge*; this is formed by the slit lamp beam. It is useful for identifying poorly demarcated Schwalbe's line. It is

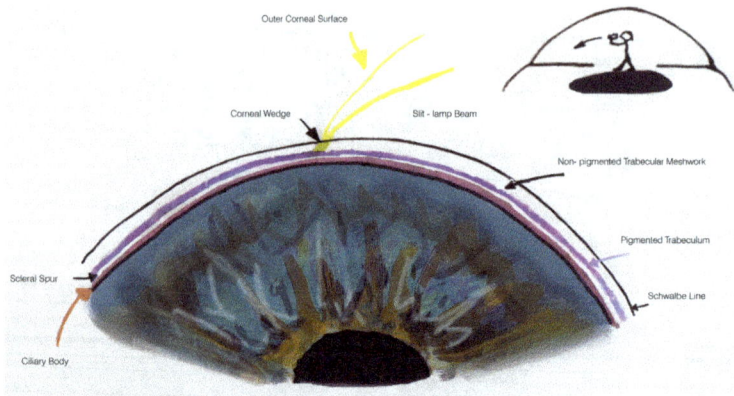

Fig. 3.10. Goniolens view.

formed by the beam reflecting from the corneal endothelium
and the beam reflecting from the corneal epithelium appearing to meet.

- *Schwalbe's line*; the termination of Descemet's Membrane
  (one of the inner layers of the cornea). This is sometimes
  pigmented and care needs to be taken not to mistake it for
  pigmented trabecular meshwork. The corneal wedge helps
  identify the structure.
- *Trabecular meshwork*; variable pigmentation from patient to
  patient.
- *Scleral Spur*; whitish termination of sclera.
- *Ciliary body*; pinkish colour only seen in the most open of
  angles.

The commonest used and easiest to learn grading system is
that of Shaffer.

- **Grade 0** Angle closed
- **Grade 1** Schwalbe line seen → Closure probable or imminent
- **Grade 2** Part of trabeculum → Closure possible
- **Grade 3** Scleral spur
- **Grade 4** Ciliary body

If the angle is closed or narrow this can increase the pressure within the eye, and therefore cause glaucomatous damage. If 180° or more of the angle is Grade 2 or less then peripheral iridotomies are indicated.

It is not only the visibility of the angle that is important in the diagnosis and management of glaucoma. The morphology and anatomical configuration of the iris is a vital component. One of the most common pathological iris configurations that relates to glaucoma is 'Plateau Iris'. Plateau iris is caused by the ciliary body being rotated slightly anteriorly, thereby causing the peripheral iris to be pushed forwards and leading to narrowing of the angle. Plateau iris can be diagnosed with a special gonioscopy technique known as indentation gonioscopy. The gonio lens used here is of a smaller size (such as the Volk G4) which allows it to rest on the cornea (no coupling agent needed) and gentle pressure to be placed on the anterior chamber to see how the iris and the angle structure respond.

Common changes seen are:

- The angle opens up completely on indentation. This indicates that the narrowing of the angle is due to thickening of the natural lens (phacomorphic).
- The angle does not open up at all. This indicates the presence of peripheral anterior synechiae.
- The iris shows a 'double-hump sign'. This indicates plateau iris. The first peripheral elevation (or 'hump') is due to the anteriorly rotated ciliary body pushing the iris forwards. This is followed by a more central dip in the iris, following which there is another elevation (or the second 'hump') due to the underlying natural lens.

Indentation gonioscopy is an advanced technique but can yield much more valuable information compared to standard gonioscopy.

However, it is essential to have comprehensive experience with standard gonioscopy (also known as non-indentation gonioscopy), before attempting this.

4

INVESTIGATIONS

Thomas Sherman

Investigations related to glaucoma are used both for diagnosis and monitoring of the condition. Investigations can be subjective, such as visual field testing; alternatively, they can be objective, where the patient is unable to influence the endpoint.

No one test is used in isolation to diagnose glaucoma, rather they are combined, allowing correlation of optic nerve function and structure.

VISUAL FIELDS

Visual field testing answers the pragmatic question of how much peripheral vision a patient has lost due to glaucoma. To understand its relevance in glaucoma there are a few basic principles and pieces of terminology to be aware of.

What is the Visual Field?

Visual field testing measures the 'hill of vision' which is a physiological model of the entire visual field. We know from basic anatomy that the macula contains the highest density of photoreceptor cells and thus has a high sensitivity to picking up fine detail. As one moves further out away from the macula to the periphery, the number of photoreceptor cells declines, so

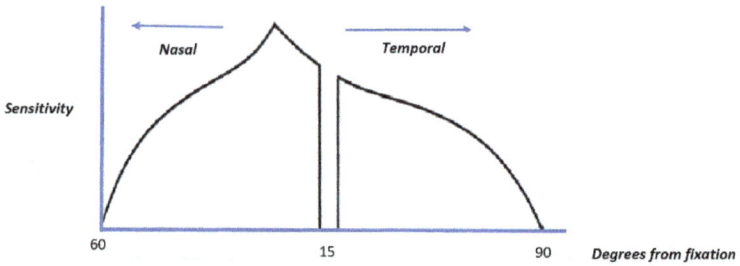

Fig. 4.1. The hill of vision showing a peak in sensitivity at the fovea and blind spot corresponding to the optic nerve head (approximately 15 degrees nasal to fovea).

too does the sensitivity of the visual field. The optic nerve has no photoreceptor cells, so it is a physiological 'blind spot' where no image can be perceived. If you were to draw this as a map it would look like Fig. 4.1.

What are the Types of Visual Field Testing?

The main type of field test used is Humphrey visual field testing. This is automated (done by a machine) and static (a light is shone in a particular spot and then appears in another spot rather than moving in gradually from peripheral to central). The opposite to this would be the Goldman visual field test which is manual (performed by a trained perimetrist) and kinetic (the target moves from peripheral to central). Naturally, kinetic perimetry has existed for longer than static perimetry, so many of the terms used in automated testing were originally used in the context of manual testing. Visual field testing can either be for each eye independently (monocular) or both eyes open (binocular). An example of binocular visual field tests is the Esterman test (Fig. 4.2) which is used in the UK to test if the visual field is sufficient for driving.

How can We Quantify the Visual Field?

At first you may think testing the visual field would be a simple case of shining a small enough spot of light in a variety

▦ OU	Suprathreshold		Esterman Binocular Suprathreshold Test	

Fixation Monitor:	Off	Stimulus:	III, White	Date:	Jun 27, 2017
Fixation Target:	Central	Background:	31.5 asb	Time:	10:17 AM
Fixation Losses:	0/0	Strategy:	Two Zone	Age:	61
False POS Errors:	0/12	Test Mode:	Single Intensity		
False NEG Errors:	0/12	Pupil Diameter:			
Test Duration:	05:50	Visual Acuity:			
Stimulus Intensity:	10dB	Rx:			

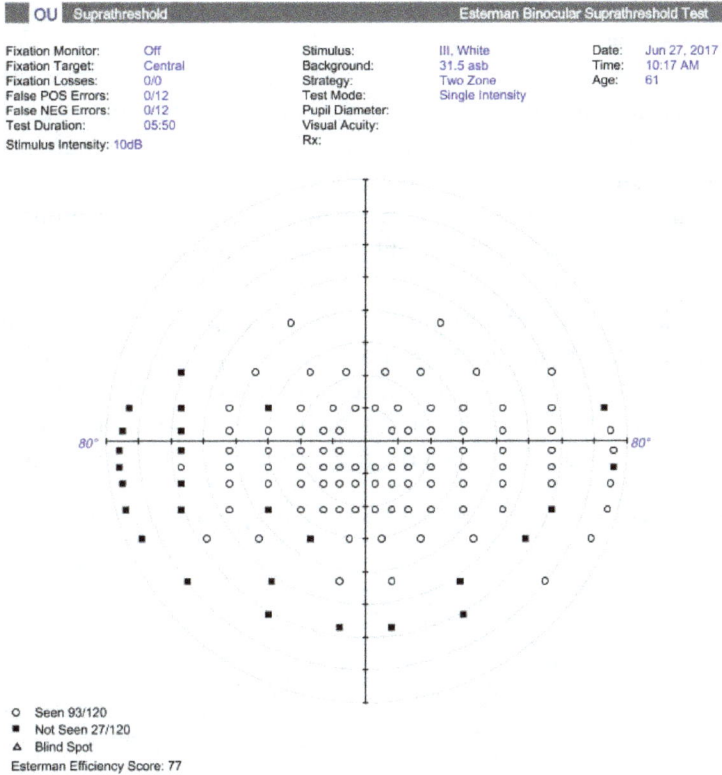

○ Seen 93/120
■ Not Seen 27/120
△ Blind Spot
Esterman Efficiency Score: 77

Fig. 4.2. Example of an Esterman visual field test. The black squares represent areas not seen. Each circle represents 10 degrees of the visual field, exact criteria for driving fitness are best reviewed at the DVLA website. This field was taken from a gentleman who was an HGV driver and did not meet the criteria for a Category II licence (as of 2018).

of positions with the patient fixing straight ahead; to produce a map of which spots are seen and which are not. However, we know the retina has different sensitivities across different areas. A sensitive area such as the macula will be able to perceive a much dimmer light than the periphery. This is the basis of Humphrey visual field testing. A stimulus of known size and brightness is attenuated (dimmed) and the amount of attenuation possible before the patient is no longer able to see the target will tell you the threshold of sensitivity.

The example below shows a typical Humphrey visual field test. A Goldman Size III stimulus (which has a standardised level of brightness and size) is used and the numeric readout shows how many decibels of attenuation are possible, which the patient reports they can see. Therefore, a high number means an area is more sensitive to detecting a stimulus. < 0 means the patient did not see the target. The background against which the lights are shone also has a standardised level of brightness (31.5 apostilbs).

It is worth mentioning that the term 'brightness' used here is a slight simplification. Brightness is a quality reported by individuals, which varies from person to person. When referring to perimetry equipment, a standardised quantity of emitted light is produced. This is termed luminous flux. Luminous flux

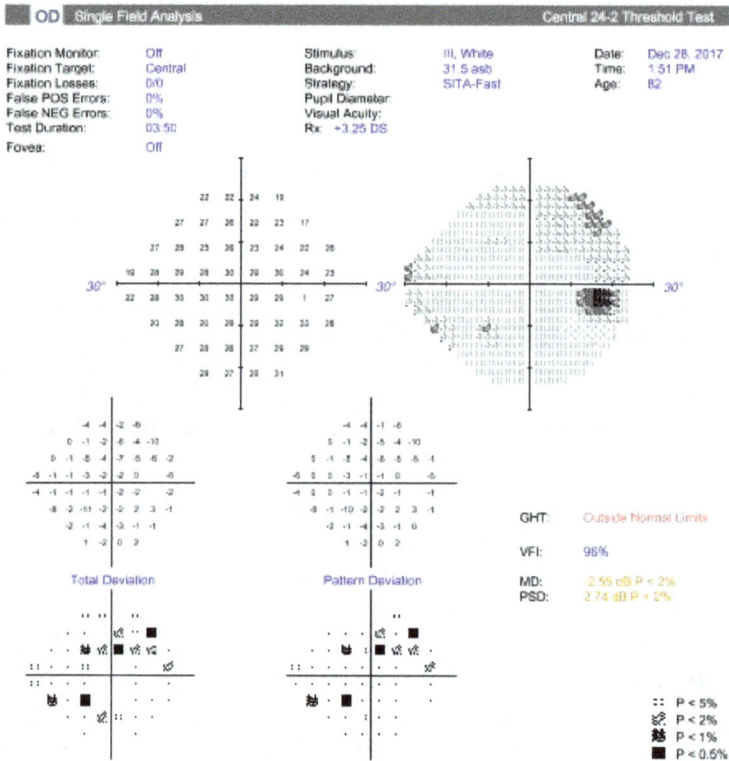

Fig. 4.3.   Humphrey visual field test.

per square metre gives the unit, apostilb. In perimetry light stimuli can be 0.08–10,000 apostilbs. To quantify this large range easily, luminous flux is expressed on a logarithmic scale, which is decibels. The total size of the scale is 51 decibels.

How is Visual Field Testing Performed?

It could potentially take hours to shine a spot of light in every area of the visual field to see if it is registered. Therefore, we need to have a set quantity of points tested at set locations across the visual field. A Humphrey field test should have 24-2, 30-2 or 10-2 displayed (there are also other less commonly used variants). The 24-2 is the standard test used for glaucoma. It measures 54 points, all separated by 6 degrees between them. The test extends 24 degrees temporally and 30 degrees nasally, to maximise the detection of early 'nasal step' defects, discussed later. A schematic for the 24-2 test is shown below.

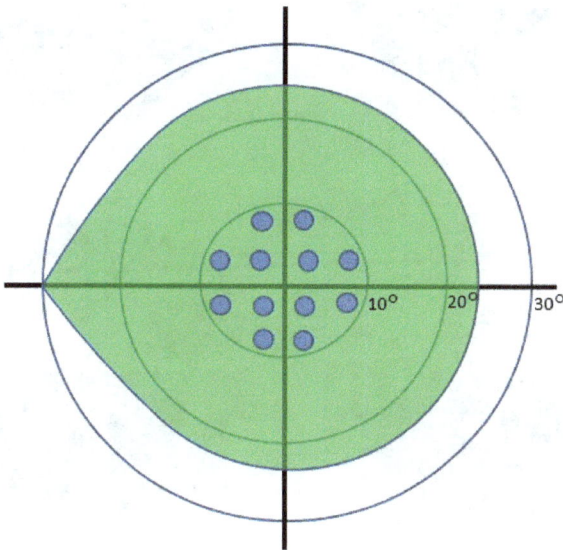

Fig. 4.4. Diagram showing the extent of a 24-2 field, this is the green shaded area. The blue dots show examples of where the points are projected, each separated by 6 degrees and spaced away from the midline, as opposed to the 24-1.

Tests ending in –1 are no longer used. They represented the first testing strategies devised and stimuli were presented on the horizontal and vertical fixation lines. This has the disadvantage of a point being potentially 'half seen' if there is a defect extending up to the midline in either direction. Thus the –2, so called as it was the second pattern of testing derived, is 3 degrees either side of the midlines (half the 6 degree gap between points).

The 30-2 tests 76 points and extends 30 degrees nasally and temporally. It is used more for neuro-ophthalmic investigation. Finally, the 10-2 measures 10 degrees nasally and temporally and uses 68 points. It is for testing the central visual field in more detail. This is often used where there is advanced visual

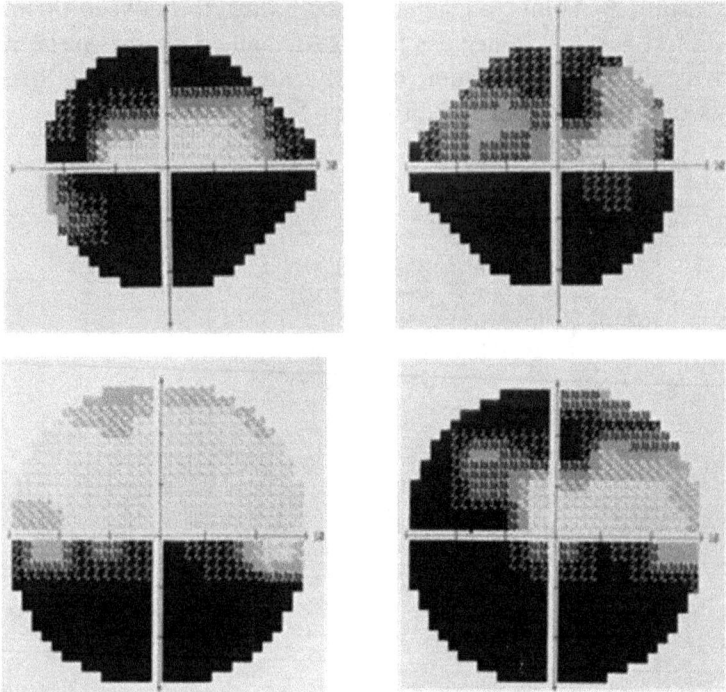

Fig. 4.5. In this case of advanced glaucoma, the central visual field looks completely blacked out on 24-2 testing (top two images- especially in the left eye) however, when a 10-2 field test is performed it can be seen that there are areas in the left eye of normal sensitivity, missed by 24-2 testing.

field loss and one wants to 'zoom in' on the central visual field, as the 24-2 test can be difficult to compare between visits when field loss is advanced.

A test programme can work out visual field thresholds on the basis of points previously presented, to reduce the time taken to complete the test. This is known as the Swedish Integrated Testing Algorithm (SITA). A variant called the SITA fast test takes around 4 minutes to perform per eye. The SITA fast programme is used at the vast majority of centres. Although there is a reduced testing time compared to SITA standard, sustained concentration is still required in addition to adequate reflex response to visual stimulus presentation. These factors mean that visual field testing will often vary between tests slightly, despite no change in visual function.

How Do I Analyse a Visual Field Test?

Armed with our understanding of the basic principles that underpin field testing, we can now begin to analyse a visual field. Here I show a printout from a Carl Zeiss Humphrey visual field test (Fig. 4.6), but most printouts are similar for different machines. We will go through how to analyse a field readout in a systematic way.

1. Demographics.
   Check the patient's details are correct
   Check the date of the test is the one you are interested in
2. Reliability indices.
   False positives
   False negatives
   Fixation losses
3. Pattern deviation map.
4. Numeric values map/greyscale.
5. Global field indices.
   Meandeviation
   VFI
   Pattern standard deviation
   Glaucoma hemifield test

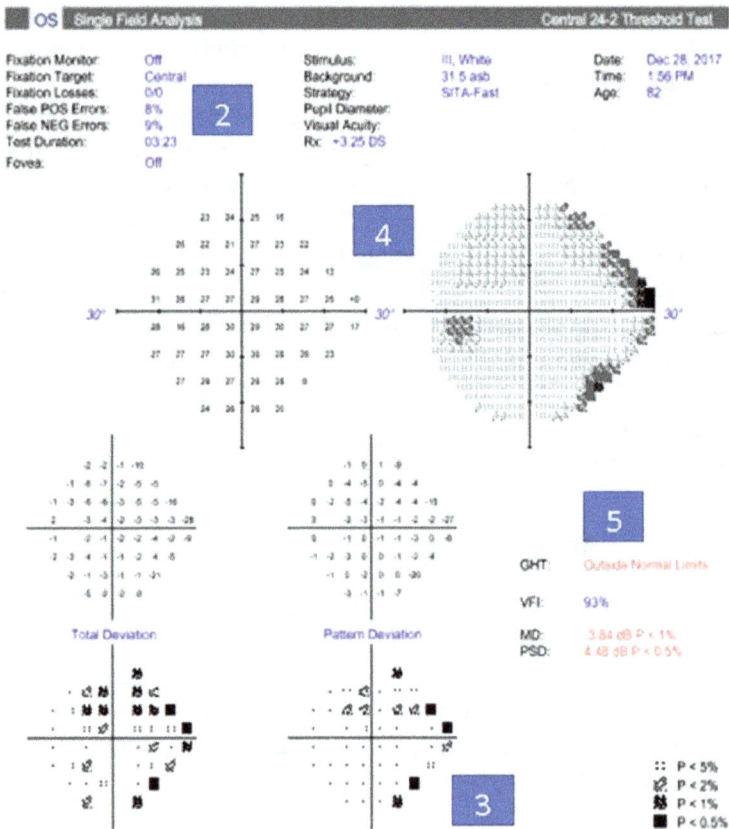

Fig. 4.6. Printout from a Humphrey visual field test (Carl Zeiss).

• **Demographics**

Always check that the correct patient's results have been uploaded, especially when the clinical picture doesn't seem to fit the test results. Another issue worth pointing out is that the testing strategy is not the same for the right and left eye. Fig. 4.7 shows the result you get if the wrong eye is selected and analysed on the field machine, in effect the blind spot is transposed to the oppose side one would expect.

• **Reliability Indices**

An accurate measure of the visual field requires a patient to maintain fixation consistently and to press the button promptly only

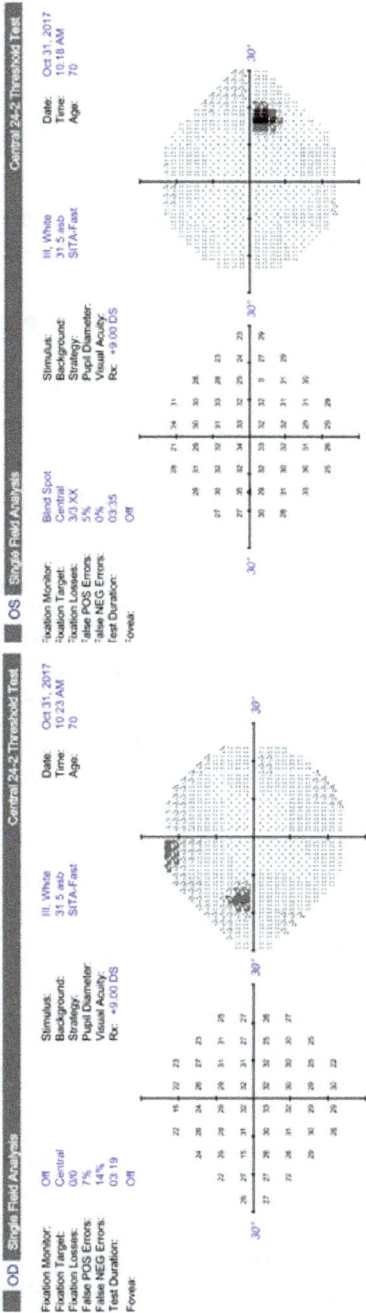

Fig. 4.7. Transposition of blind spot when wrong eye selected on field machine. Note that the test is still relatively 'accurate' on reliability parameters.

when a target is seen. Unfortunately, this degree of sustained concentration and fast reaction can prove challenging, especially for elderly patients or those with cognitive impairment. This always has to be borne in mind when requesting field tests.

To judge a test's reliability there are 4 parameters available. The false positive rate is a percentage of the number of times the patient acknowledged the presence of a stimulus when none was presented. This often happens if there is a sustained interval of time between points presented as patients can feel they 'should be seeing something'. A false positive rate of 15% or more invalidates the field test.

It is worth pointing out to patients with a high false positive rate that occasionally the visual field machine makes a noise which usually accompanies the stimulus appearing. However, on occasion it will make the noise but no light appears. The patient may click the button when they hear the noise in error. It is not 'cheating' to inform them of this and ask them to only press the button when they see a light, even if it seems one has not appeared for a long time. Another issue is that patients can take exception to being told their hard work in the field testing machine was 'unreliable', so an empathetic approach in counselling the patient on how to do the test is essential. Phrases such as 'trigger happy' are not received well, especially if you work in a military hospital!

The other reliability indices carry less weight than the false positive rate. One will often see false negative rates of 10% or so even in reliable field tests. A false negative occurs when a patient does not acknowledge the stimulus, despite that stimulus previously being presented at the same area at a less attenuated level. 'False negative' results can also result if a patient briefly lost fixation and so a different area is tested. Additionally, when there is damage to the nerve fibre layer, visual field thresholds can be variable. This makes it hard to ascribe a value of a false negative that would invalidate the test, although ones in excess of 20% generally confer poor reliability.

Fixation losses can register at a higher rate than actually occurred, the perimetrist supervising the test will often be able

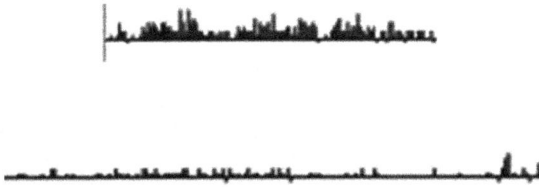

Fig. 4.8. An erratic gaze trace shown above, and a more even, sustained, gaze shown below.

to comment on whether fixation was actually lost or not as it can easily be seen when a patient is looking around. Finally, the gaze tracker can be used to qualitatively judge how much a patient was looking around. Fig. 4.8 shows some examples of good fixation and erratic eye movements.

- **Total/Pattern Deviation Maps**

The total deviation map shows areas that are of reduced threshold sensitivity compared to what would be expected for a healthy age matched individual. This goes some way to accounting for natural, age related attrition of optic nerve function. The map has 4 scales of probability, indicated by the pattern of the square. The lower the number, the greater the probability that the result seen at that point is pathological. For example a dotted square (< 5%) means 95% of age adjusted test subjects scored a higher value than the patient's score. A black square means 99.5% of participants scored higher, making the probability that the deviation is simply a variant of normal extremely unlikely.

The other small map using the same scale is the pattern deviation. A neat definition of pattern deviation is 'the adjustment of the visual field test to account for the overall hill of vision'. If a patient has a cataract, or a dry corneal surface, the sensitivity threshold will be globally reduced, as less light enters the eye. However, we are not interested in using field tests to judge if someone has a cataract, we are interested in whether there are discrete areas of field loss due to nerve fibre loss in that area. This is what the pattern deviation will display, as it adjusts for the overall decreases in sensitivity.

- **Greyscale Map**

The two large maps at the top of the field printout are in essence the 'raw data' of the visual field test from which the lower two map results are calculated. The map on the left is a numeric map of how many decibels of attenuation were achieved. It is an often overlooked area on the field printout when scanning through. However, it can give useful information. For example, where someone has a reading of more than 40dB of attenuation, the result is exceedingly likely to be a false positive, thus one can use the map to localise areas of false positives.

Perhaps a more practical use is in differentiating neurological from glaucomatous defects. In glaucoma, nerve fibres are steadily lost from the superior and inferior radiations from the macula. What one often sees is a graded, spreading reduction in level of attenuation across the affected area. Whereas in a neurological defect, or a vascular occlusive event such as a retinal artery occlusion, there will be a sharp delineation. One area might read 25, then immediately next to it is an area < 0. A neurological defect also should respect the vertical midline, whereas the glaucomatous defect respects the horizontal midline. The greyscale is just a graphical depiction of this information. It is a useful 'at a glance' guide to the patient's threshold sensitivities across their visual field. The darker colours indicate a lower sensitivity than lighter colours. The problem with the greyscale is that it is not age matched and does not account for the overall hill of vision in the way that the pattern deviation does.

- **Global Field Indices**

The mean deviation can be quantified as an average of the patient's overall departure from the age adjusted level of sensitivity. A mean deviation of 0 means they are at the expected level of threshold sensitivity, a value beyond −2dB suggests a pathological decrease and a positive value shows the patient has a better than expected level of visual field sensitivity. There is no formal range but a value of up to or beyond −12dB indicates severe visual field loss. This mean deviation can be plotted on a graph to analyse progression of glaucoma over time, which is detailed later.

The pattern standard deviation score numerically quantifies how much variation there is over the entire visual field. It is measured by calculating how much a patient's threshold departs from the age expected value for each individual point. Therefore, if a field is uniformly depressed, there will be a low PSD. If there is a focal defect (such as in glaucoma) the PSD will be higher (it can be described as a numerical representation of the Pattern Deviation map mentioned earlier).

The visual field index is an index similar to the mean deviation, but weighted to the central points of the visual field and quantified on a percentage scale rather than dB. Software exists that can give some idea as to the rate of glaucomatous field progression. Fig. 4.9 is an example of the GPA (glaucoma progression analysis), which is incorporated into the Carl Zeiss Humphrey visual field machine. A minimum of 5 reliable visual fields are required before this chart can be plotted, it is then able to plot a chart on the basis of VFI results and can extrapolate to demonstrate the rate of visual field loss (blue line). The below examples show the utility of this measure.

Figure 4.9 shows an advanced defect that is stable, as the blue line does not drop below around 60% VFI. Note that although the fields are accurate (low false positive and negative values) there is too wide a confidence interval to plot an extrapolation curve, detailed later. Generally, a confidence interval of less than +/–2.5% is needed for an accurate extrapolation. At the bottom of the GPA printout is a map (far right) that demonstrates the points of the visual field where progression is seen. The software chooses a suitably accurate baseline visual field test and then compares subsequent tests to this. A white triangle shows that statistically significant progression has been noted on one occasion. However, the clinical significance that can be attached to this is often uncertain, due to inter-test variability. Where the same area is continually flagged as showing deterioration, the significance becomes more certain, indicated by a black triangle. The 'out of range' mark means that the GPA could not determine if the change encountered was

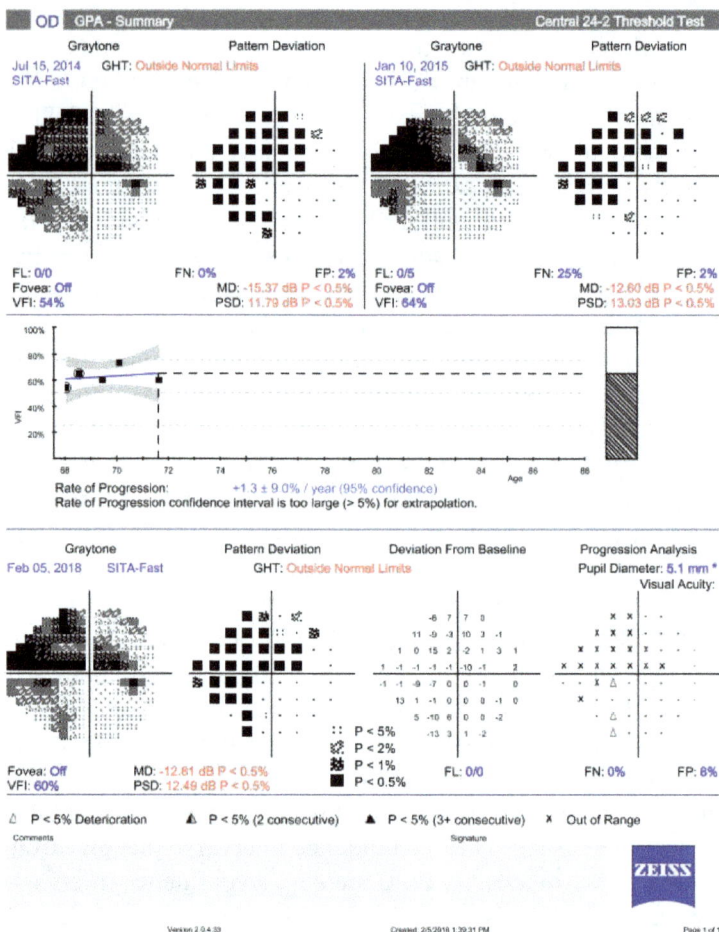

Fig. 4.9. Example GPA printout.

significant. This typically occurs if the VFI score on the latest field was higher than the baseline (i.e. a theoretical 'improvement' in the field) or if there was already a deep defect at baseline. The black dots represent areas of no significant change.

Figure 4.10 shows a rapidly progressing field defect. Here, a narrower confidence interval means that extrapolation line can be plotted. In this case the extrapolation extends for the next 4 years, as indicated by the bar chart at the side of the

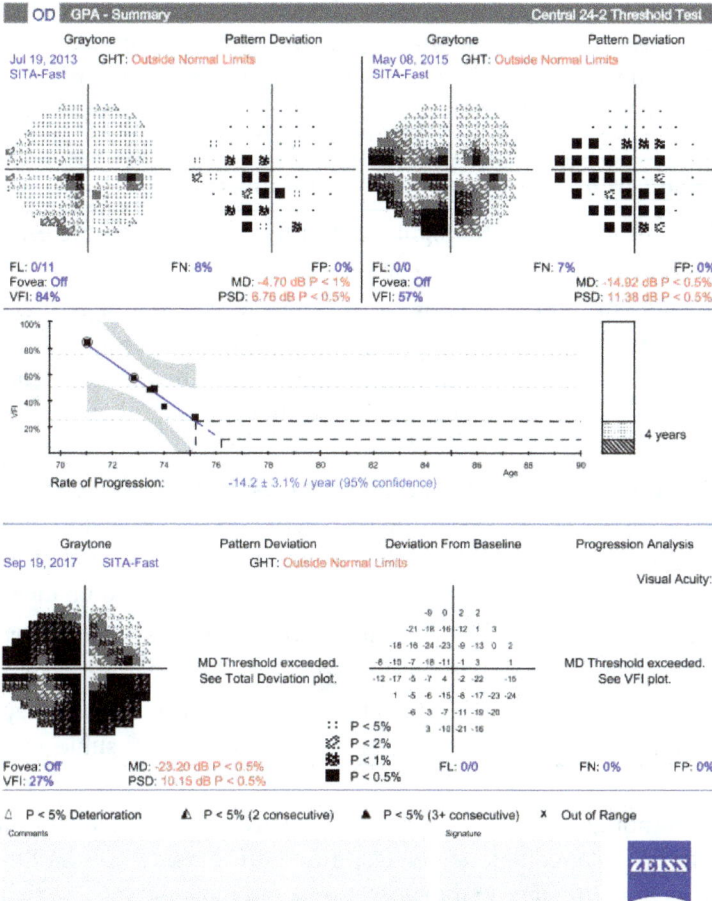

Fig. 4.10. Example GPA printout.

progression chart. The maximum duration of time that can be extrapolated is 5 years. This is an example of a case that will likely need surgical intervention to achieve a sufficient control of intraocular pressure, providing there is not an alternative explanation for visual field compromise.

Finally, the Glaucoma Hemifield Test (GHT) attempts to alert the clinician to a potential diagnosis of glaucoma for new cases. It works on the principle that glaucoma will cause asymmetric damage to the papillomacular bundle either side of the horizontal meridian. It compares five pre-defined areas in one hemifield against the other, to give one of five different outcomes listed below.

Result from GHT	Implication
Within normal limits	No significant difference between zones.
Outside normal limits	One or more zones in one hemifield differ to a statistically significant extent compared to the other hemifield. The p value is < 0.01 indicating this is very unlikely due to chance.
Borderline	One or more zones show a statistically significant difference however the p value is higher at < 0.03, so a greater probability this could be due to chance.
General Depression	Stimulus area scores are so low that they occur only in 0.5% of normal subjects.
Abnormally high sensitivity	Stimulus area scores are so high that they occur only in 0.5% of normal subjects.

Although the GHT has a high sensitivity and specificity for detecting glaucomatous defects, a one off 'outside normal limits' is not sufficient to diagnose glaucoma in isolation. The field must be interpreted in the context of the whole clinical picture.

Visual Field Defects

One of the crucial elements of glaucoma management is ensuring that the diagnosis is made accurately, and that one is not missing a potentially life-threatening neuro-ophthalmic problem. The key rule in ensuring that diagnosis is accurate is that the disc must match the fields. For example, a superior arcuate defect should accompany an inferior nerve fibre layer defect. If the disc does not match the expected field defect then one should consider an MRI scan of the head and orbits to image for a lesion along the visual pathway. The typical early visual defect is a nasal step (Fig. 4.11).

Another field defect that can be seen is a paracentral scotoma. This tends to be seen particularly in normotension glaucoma. Although small, it can be particularly problematic as it may be visually symptomatic and can have implications for driving if there are symmetric changes in both eyes. Fig. 4.12 demonstrates such a scotoma.

The early field defects can then progress to arcuate changes, which can be superior or inferior. Further progression beyond

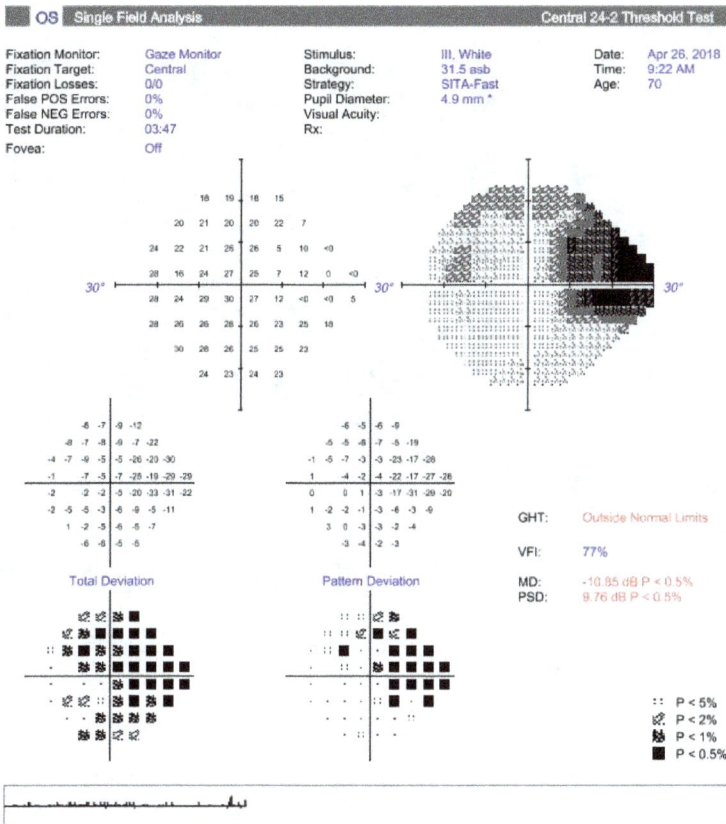

Fig. 4.11. A nasal step defect.

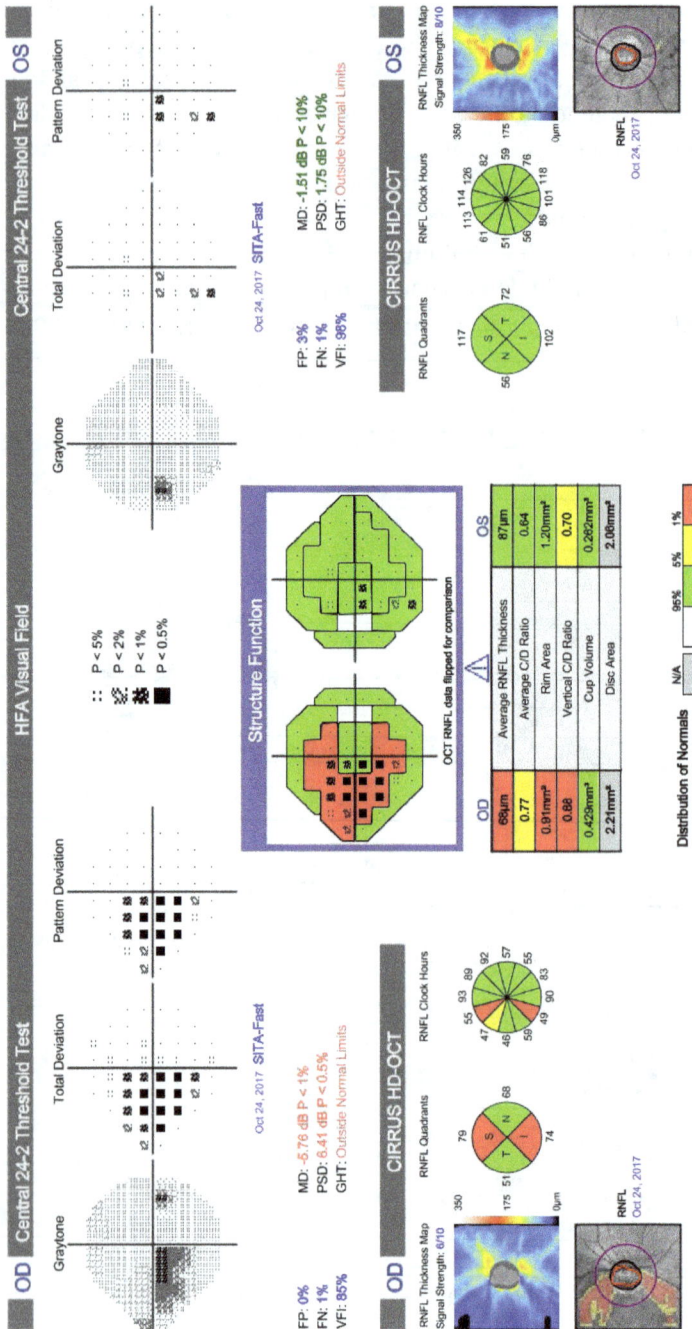

Fig. 4.12. A structure-function printout that maps a paracentral inferior defect in the right eye with a corresponding nerve fibre defect (the central map shows that the red areas of nerve fibre loss match up perfectly to the scotoma).

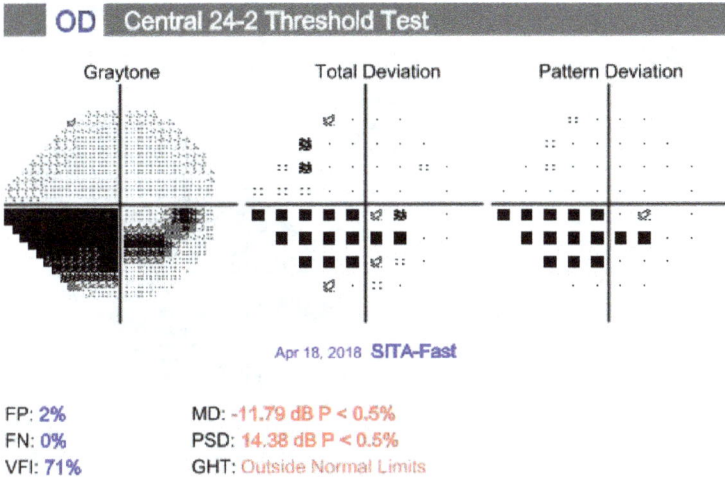

OD Central 24-2 Threshold Test

Graytone | Total Deviation | Pattern Deviation

Apr 18, 2018 **SITA-Fast**

FP: **2%**
FN: **0%**
VFI: **71%**

MD: **-11.79 dB P < 0.5%**
PSD: **14.38 dB P < 0.5%**
GHT: Outside Normal Limits

Fig. 4.13. An example of an inferior arcuate scotoma progressing into an altitudinal defect nasally.

this leads to an altitudinal field defect that respects the horizontal midline (Fig. 4.13).

Advanced visual field loss can then follow (Fig. 4.14). Often the central field is relatively spared in glaucoma until very late stage disease. As previously mentioned, a 10-2 Humphrey visual field test is useful for monitoring the central visual field, as this can be difficult using a 24-2.

Visual Fields in Context

The problem with visual field testing is its potentially wide variability between visits. It gives the impression of being a very quantitative and exact measure of visual field function, in reality there is a lot of 'noise' related to the test. This can be due to a multitude of patient related factors, such as fatigue and distraction. The art of glaucoma involves triangulating field results with the intraocular pressure, structural disc changes, how invasive the next step of intervention is and the patient's overall health. For example, if a progressing field means changing someone's drop, this may not be as significant

OD Single Field Analysis   Central 24-2 Threshold Test

Fixation Monitor: Off   Stimulus: III, White   Date: Sep 19, 2017
Fixation Target: Central   Background: 31.5 asb   Time: 9:47 AM
Fixation Losses: 0/0   Strategy: SITA-Fast   Age: 75
False POS Errors: 0%   Pupil Diameter:
False NEG Errors: 0%   Visual Acuity:
Test Duration: 04:49   Rx: +2.75 DC X 171
Fovea: Off

```
              11  22 | 22  21
          2    4   7 | 9  22  24
      <0   4   0  <0 | 12   8  22  23
  <0  <0  11  <0  <0 | 23  13  <0  24
30°<0 <0  17  <0  <0 | 22   0  <0   5    30°                    30°
      13  17  16  <0 | <0   0   0  <0
           8   3   0 | <0  <0   2
               4  <0 | <0   2
```

```
         -15  -4 | -4  -4
     -26 -25 -21 |-19  -6  -3
  -30 -25 -30 -32 |-18 -24  -7  -4
-26 -31 -19 -33 -34 | -8 -16      -5              MD Threshold exceeded.
-26 -31 -14 -34 -34 |-10 -31      -24             See Total Deviation plot.
 -15 -13 -15 -34 |-33 -31 -30 -31
     -21 -27 -30 |-32 -32 -27                     GHT:    Outside Normal Limits
          -24 -31 |-31 -27
                                                  VFI:    27%
         Total Deviation              Pattern Deviation    MD:     -23.20 dB P < 0.5%
                                                  PSD:    10.15 dB P < 0.5%
```

MD Threshold exceeded.
See Total Deviation plot.

```
                           ::   P < 5%
                           ⌀    P < 2%
                           ▨    P < 1%
                           ■    P < 0.5%
```

Comments   Signature

ZEISS

HFA II - 740 9573/5.0   Version 2.0.4.33   Created: 9/19/2017 9:55:42 AM   Page 1 of 1

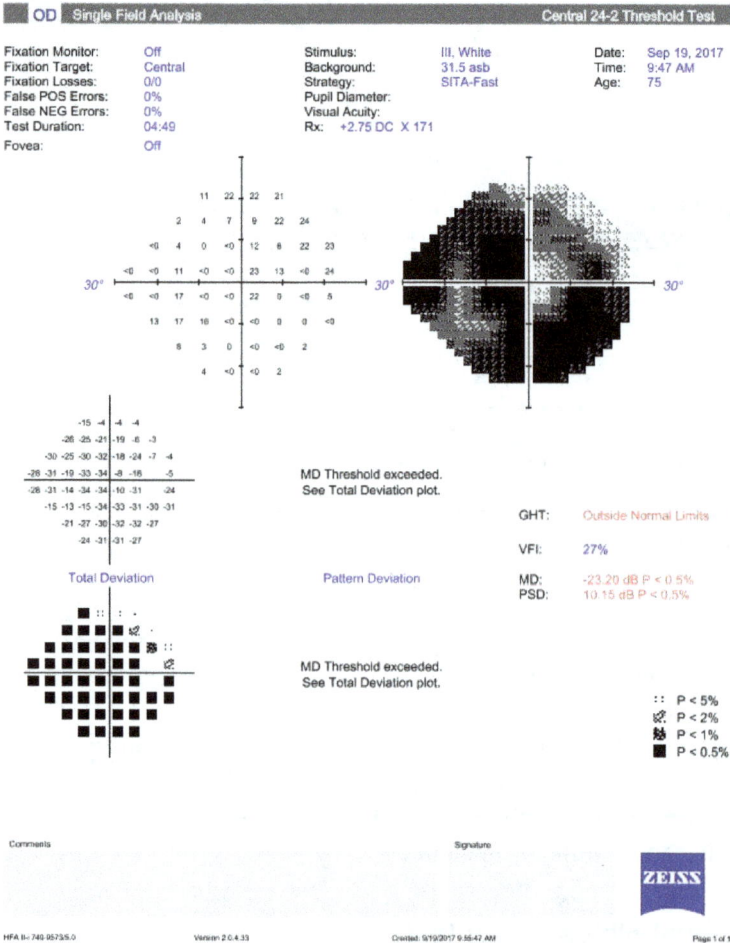

Fig. 4.14. Advanced visual field loss, note that the pattern deviation map often cannot be plotted when defects reach this level of severity. Patients may still have a relatively preserved acuity as there is a central area of sparing, however this level of field defect is almost invariably symptomatic.

a leap as performing drainage surgery. In some cases, even despite good intraocular pressure control, glaucomatous field loss can continue to deteriorate.

OPTICAL COHERENCE TOMOGRAPHY (OCT)

Visual fields tell us about optic nerve function, however assessing optic nerve structure is also important. OCT is now widely used to provide optic nerve head imaging, having historically been used to provide detailed images of the macula. There are many different manufacturers of OCT machines however all machines use a similar principle for scanning and a similar printout for analysis. Here I have shown a variety of readouts from the Zeiss and Topcon devices.

How Does OCT Scanning Work?

OCT allows high-resolution cross-sectional (tomographic) images of the retina and optic disc to be obtained in a non-invasive manner. It works by measuring the properties of light waves reflected from tissue (similar to sound wave measurements in ultrasonography). However, the utilization of light instead of sound presents a technical challenge. The speed of light makes direct measurements on the reflected waves impossible. In OCT systems, this hurdle is overcome through the use of a technique called interferometry. In interferometry, a beam of light is divided into a measuring beam and a reference beam. The reconvergence of light reflected from the tissue of interest and light reflected from a reference path produces characteristic patterns of interference that are dependent on the mismatch between the reflected waves (Fig. 4.15). Because the time delay and amplitude of one of the waves (i.e., the reference path) is known, the time delay and intensity of light returning from the sample tissue may then be extracted from the interference pattern. A two-dimensional or three-dimensional image of the retina and optic disc is then created.

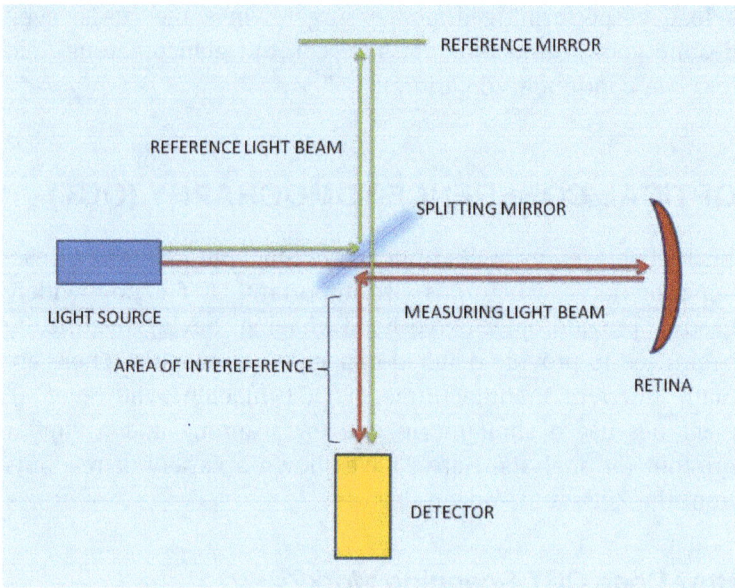

Fig. 4.15. Schematic diagram of a Michelson interferometer demonstrating the principle of optical coherence tomography.

How to Analyse an OCT Printout

1. Check demographics and date of scan.
2. Check reliability index.
3. Compare heat maps/deviation maps.
4. Look at nerve fibre layer parameters.
5. Look at nerve fibre layer sectoral map.

Reliability Index

Located at the top of the printout, this quantifies the strength of the signal received by the transducer. It can be affected by cataract and other sources of ocular media opacity, e.g., corneal scarring. Changes to the retina around the optic disc or macula, such as epiretinal membrane can also affect reliability of OCT readings. The manufacturers of the Zeiss machine label scans with a score of 6/10 or more as being reliable. On the Topcon device the reliability index is given a score that should be over 40. The other way to judge if a scan is reliable is to ensure that the images taken are crisp, with no signs of blink artefact (Fig. 4.16) and that a clear picture of the optic nerve head is visible.

Although not included in the reliability index, another factor that can markedly affect scan results is the placement of the calculation circle. Most machines contain software that will

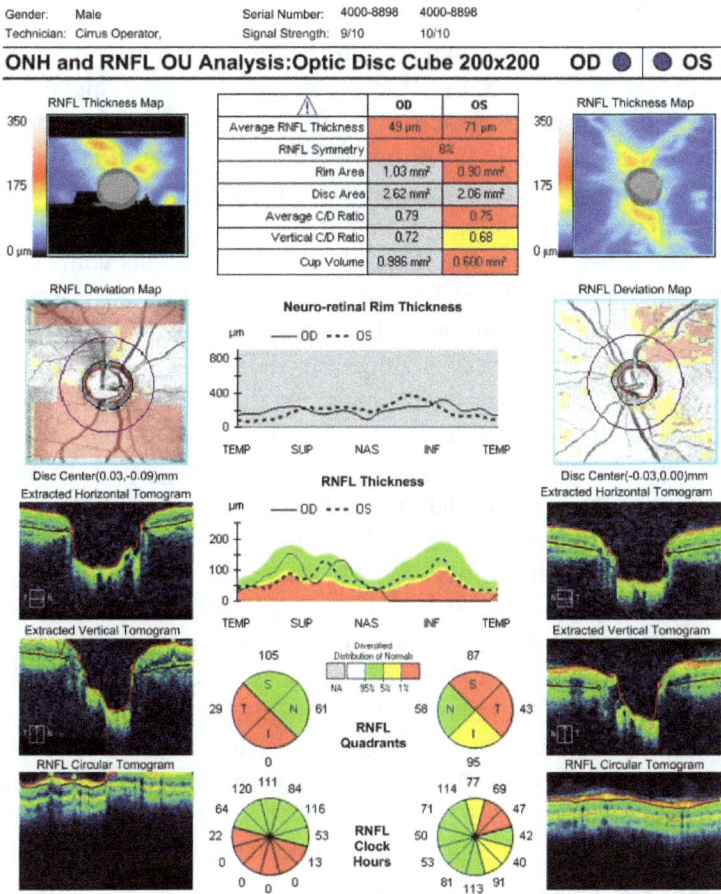

Fig. 4.16. Blink artefact; an incomplete scan of the right eye inferior nerve fibre layer results in false readings of 0 microns.

automatically detect the optic disc and centre a circle around it from which the calculations of nerve fibre layer thickness are measured. However, it is possible to manually adjust the placement of this circle as well. It is important to be aware that readings taken off-centre will not be reliable. Additionally, optic discs that are tilted (where the optic nerve insertion into the globe is oblique) cannot be reliably analysed.

Heat Maps/Deviation Maps

The top retinal nerve fibre layer (RNFL) thickness map is a graphical depiction of the absolute nerve fibre layer thickness. The yellow to white colours indicate a thicker nerve fibre layer and bluer colours indicate nerve fibre layer loss. Examining nerve fibre layer defects can be difficult clinically, however the OCT makes these changes far more obvious.

The other map is the RNFL deviation map. This compares the nerve fibre layer thickness values obtained to those stored in the normative database of the device. The resulting map has a yellow or red overlay highlighting the areas of nerve fibre layer loss. The normative database for the Zeiss machine is a collection of 284 individual's scans aged between 19 and 84. An appropriate age adjusted sample is then compared to the patient's scan. This is what produces the red and yellow and for the various parameters. A similar database also exists for the Topcon device and other devices. There are slightly different numbers of patients with different age distributions, which means readings between machines are not comparable. The normative databases also do not include individuals under 19 years old and exclude individuals with extremes of refractive status. For example, the Zeiss device excludes patients beyond −12 diopters and above +8 diopters. There are also differences between ethnicities in terms of RNFL. Although normative databases are ethnically diverse, they still remain predominantly composed of Caucasians.

Numeric Data

The numeric data provided as part of the disc OCT printout is a combination of measurements of the optic nerve head and thickness of the nerve fibre layer. The nerve fibre layer measurements are taken from a calculation circle that is shown below in purple, the optic nerve head measurements are derived from the black and red outlines projected over the disc scan. The disc is detected by software built into the device but can be manually altered. This then can be compared to the normative database. Grey shaded boxes appear where there is no normative database to compare with, which is always the case for disc area. Generally, the most commonly reviewed parameter is that of average RNFL thickness. With age and increasing glaucomatous damage, this thins over time. Progression of glaucoma as measured on OCT is discussed later.

The disc measurements are less commonly used in clinical practice, as it is possible to measure the size of the disc and CDR using clinical examination techniques. Generally, once one is experienced in examining discs, it becomes preferable to use one's own sense of what the CDR is, rather than relying on OCT.

Nerve Fibre Layer Sectoral Map

The exact areas affected by RNFL thinning can be anatomically detailed using the central column of maps. In Figure 4.18 the right eye has an inferior nerve fibre layer defect, which is very prominent on the heat map, and alongside which the inferior RNFL quadrant is markedly thin too. This is then further subdivided into individual clock hours, which allows one to keep track of exact areas of thinning with time. In glaucoma the superior and inferior RNFL quadrants are usually involved first.

The table below shows values taken from Carl Zeiss' instructions for interpreting disc OCTs. In this example, 95% of values for 69 year old patients in the normative database fall within the reported ranges. Note how they follow the ISNT rule.

Technician: Signal Strength: 9/10   9/10

ONH and RNFL OU Analysis:Optic Disc Cube 200x200   OD ● | ● OS

	OD	OS
Average RNFL Thickness	49 µm	69 µm
RNFL Symmetry	18%	
Rim Area	0.46 mm²	0.90 mm²
Disc Area	1.47 mm²	1.63 mm²
Average C/D Ratio	0.83	0.57
Vertical C/D Ratio	0.87	0.51
Cup Volume	0.394 mm³	0.226 mm³

RNFL Thickness Map

RNFL Deviation Map

Disc Center(-0.03,0.03)mm
Extracted Horizontal Tomogram

Extracted Vertical Tomogram

RNFL Circular Tomogram

Neuro-retinal Rim Thickness

— OD - - - OS

RNFL Thickness

— OD - - - OS

Disc Center(0.18,0.15)mm
Extracted Horizontal Tomogram

RNFL Quadrants

RNFL Clock Hours

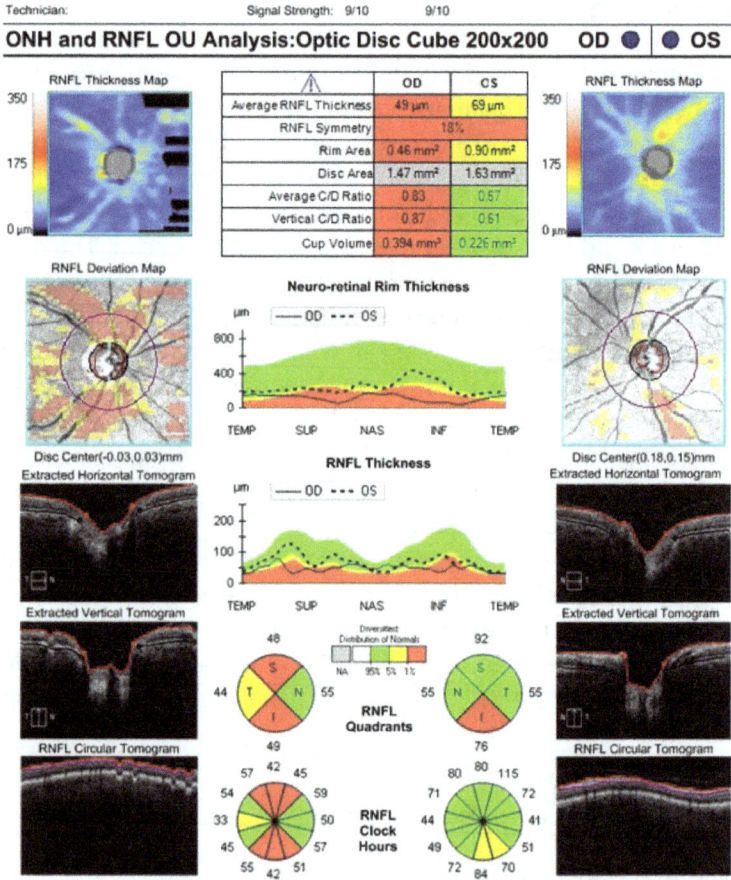

Fig. 4.17. The colour bar shows that all RNFL measurements are within the thinnest 1% of individuals assessed for the right eye, and therefore likely to be abnormal. The average cup:disc ratio for the left eye is within the 90% thickness range of cases (95% to 5%) and the left average RNFL is within the thinnest 5% of cases, so may be abnormal. Where the thickness is greater than the 95% upper limit it is detailed in white. This can flag up that the disc is swollen but is also frequently seen in healthy normal discs.

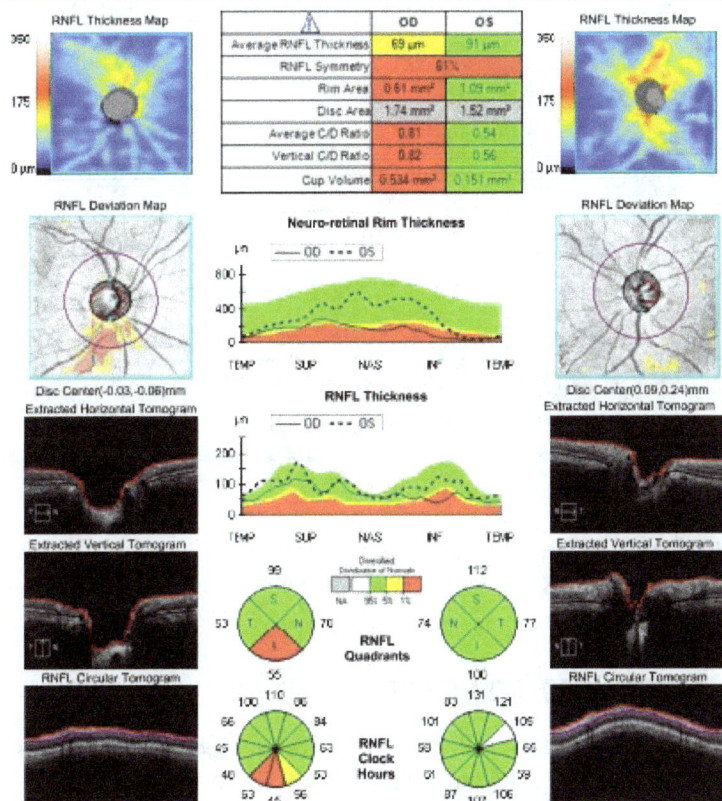

ONH and RNFL OU Analysis:Optic Disc Cube 200x200   OD ● | ● OS

	OD	OS
Average RNFL Thickness	69 µm	91 µm
RNFL Symmetry	61%	
Rim Area	0.61 mm²	1.09 mm²
Disc Area	1.74 mm²	1.52 mm²
Average C/D Ratio	0.81	0.54
Vertical C/D Ratio	0.82	0.56
Cup Volume	0.534 mm³	0.151 mm³

Fig. 4.18.

	Normal Range (microns)
Inferior	89.4–138.3
Superior	88.9–136.7
Nasal	50.0–86.2
Temporal	45.1–82.2

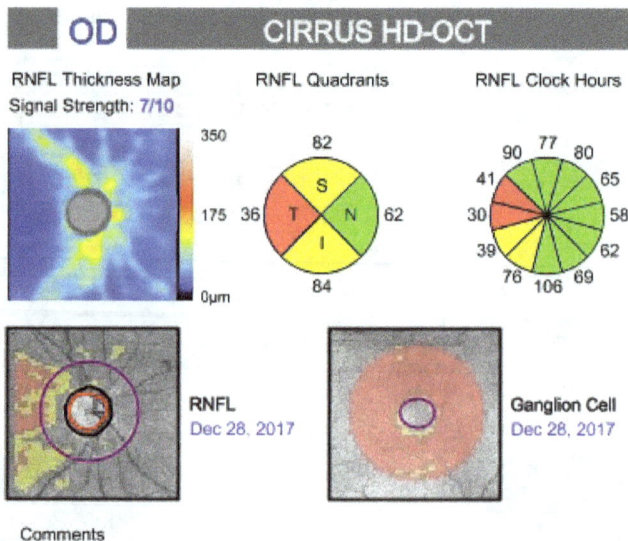

Fig. 4.19. OCT of disc and macula showing a ganglion cell layer defect in keeping with Retinal Nerve Fibre Layer thinning and a cupped optic disc.

Macular Ganglion Cell Layer Imaging

OCT can also be used to measure RNFL and ganglion cell layer health around the macula. These fibres are often the first to be affected in glaucoma (Fig. 4.19).

Progression of Glaucoma on OCT Scanning

Examining the RNFL for evidence of progression is still a relatively emerging area in glaucoma. One issue is separating what a pathological rate of RNFL loss is versus the normal expected decline in RNFL thickness with age. There have been multiple studies looking at what this rate should be. A variety of figures ranging from –0.19 microns/year to –0.52 microns/year have been demonstrated. Additionally, the rate of loss is affected by the initial baseline thickness of the RNFL, a steeper decline is noted where this value is initially higher. Different refractive states have different baseline RNFL thicknesses, with myopes tending to have thinner values. It is also worth bearing in mind that each quadrant of the optic nerve head experiences age-related loss at different rates.

Both Topcon and Zeiss machines have software that can be used to plot the changes in average RNFL thickness over time for individual patients. This is similar to the GPA function used for visual field testing. The advantage here is that RNFL changes may precede visual field loss. For pre-perimetric glaucoma, monitoring RNFL thickness will give an idea as to whether the disease is progressive or stable, hopefully before visual field loss is incurred. However, there are drawbacks. It is difficult to precisely define the relationship between loss of RNFL on OCT and visual field loss. It is therefore challenging to strike a balance between providing overly invasive measures of intraocular pressure control, versus delay in treatment, relying only on disc OCT. A further problem linked to this ambiguity about the precise relationship between RNFL thickness and visual field loss is seen in advanced glaucoma. A patient's vision may still be relatively preserved despite advanced RNFL loss on OCT. The loss may be at such a level that OCT scans struggle to reliably measure the RNFL thickness accurately between visits. This is a so called 'floor effect'. The reason this floor effect occurs is that blood vessels and supportive structures in the optic nerve head remain even after neural tissue has been lost. The OCT also struggles to accurately segment tissue once a critical point is reached, contributing to the floor effect. There are varying reports as to the precise thickness at which the floor effect occurs, it is usually at around 53 micrometres but can be less. This is important to be aware of as the OCT may show that there is no further progression of RNFL thinning, whilst the visual field may continue to deteriorate. Overall, OCT can offer an objective measure of progression, but the significance of results can be difficult to contextualise. Generally speaking, loss of more than 2 microns per year is likely to indicate pathology, as this falls outside the normal age-related rates of RNFL loss for the majority of studies. However, the visual significance of this remains uncertain. Although 'progression' may be flagged up, this doesn't always necessitate escalation to the next step of glaucoma management, but must be set in context of the individual patient.

ANTERIOR CHAMBER IMAGING

Increasingly, anterior chamber imaging is being used to achieve a useful documentations of angle status, as well as offering the advantage of a transverse section through the anterior chamber rather than looking at the angle 'straight on' in a coronal plane, as is done with gonioscopy. However, these techniques will never replace gonioscopy, which has the potential to examine angle features not yet easily identified on anterior segment imaging.

Anterior Chamber Angle OCT

Just as OCT has been used to image the macula and optic nerve, it can provide a detailed picture of the anterior chamber angle. There are different images that can be acquired using OCT. The main ones used are a single cross-sectional scan across the eye or a 5-line raster scan of the nasal and temporal angles. A raster simply refers to a rectangular matrix of pixels arranged in lines. In either format, an important landmark to identify is the scleral spur. This appears as the most anterior protrusion of the sclera that can be identified. Above this landmark is the trabeculum (Fig. 4.20). There are various measurements that can be taken, all of which utilise the scleral spur as a landmark to measure against. These are aimed at providing a quantitative measure of how open or closed the angle is. At the time of writing, a normative database adjusted for each ethnicity has yet to be established, so these measurements are mostly used academically. Currently, the use of anterior segment OCT in clinical practice is more qualitative than quantitative. It is easy to tell the difference between a clearly open angle and one that is closed. For example, in Figure 4.21 one can see how there is an open angle with no signs of iris apposition to the trabeculum.

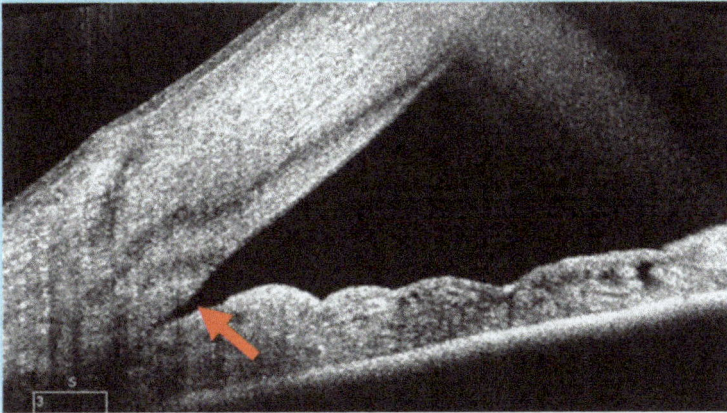

Fig. 4.20. An inwards deflection is seen (red arrow) corresponding to the scleral spur. The trabeculum is anterior to this.

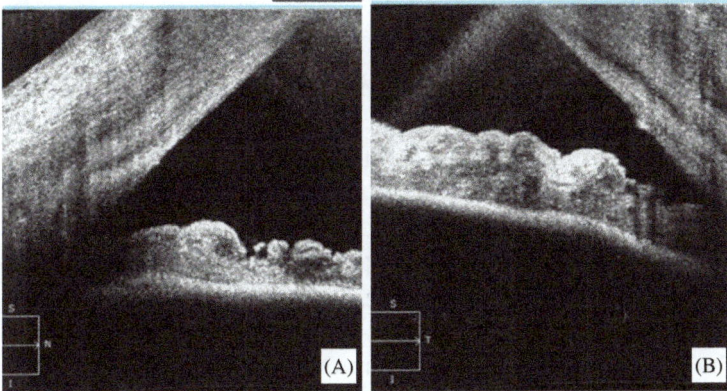

Fig. 4.21. A 5-line raster angle OCT in a pseudophakic patient showing an open angle (A). This is contrasted with the fellow eye that has a moderate amount of cataract (B). Although the angle was still open, it can be appreciated that the angle is slightly shallower as an effect of the thicker lens.

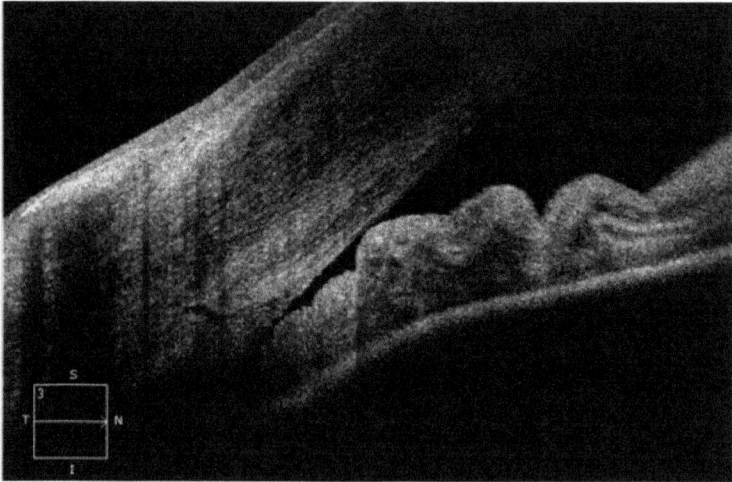

Fig. 4.22. A 5-line raster angle OCT taken from a patient with acute angle closure glaucoma in their right eye. There is evidence of iridotrabecular contact.

In Fig. 4.22, one can see how the iris abuts the trabecular face in a closed angle. The more challenging cases are those that are intermediate between these two extremes. Such cases illustrate the value of retaining skills in gonioscopy whilst this imaging technique is researched further.

Anterior segment OCT is still evolving as a technique for evaluating the anterior chamber, as such the limitations it carries centre around uncertainty as to which parameters provide the most clinically useful measurements. The other limitation linked to this is the difficulty in consistently identifying the important landmark of the scleral spur, with even experienced specialists finding this challenging. The technique itself does have the ability to identify angle structures with high resolution, however OCT is not able to visualise beyond the iris to see the ciliary body, as the iris absorbs the light signal. This is the major limitation of OCT compared to ultrasound biomicroscopy. Furthermore, artefacts can be seen when the scan is not properly centred, as seen in Fig. 4.23, where a 'shadow' of the cornea crosses the main image. Additionally, the point

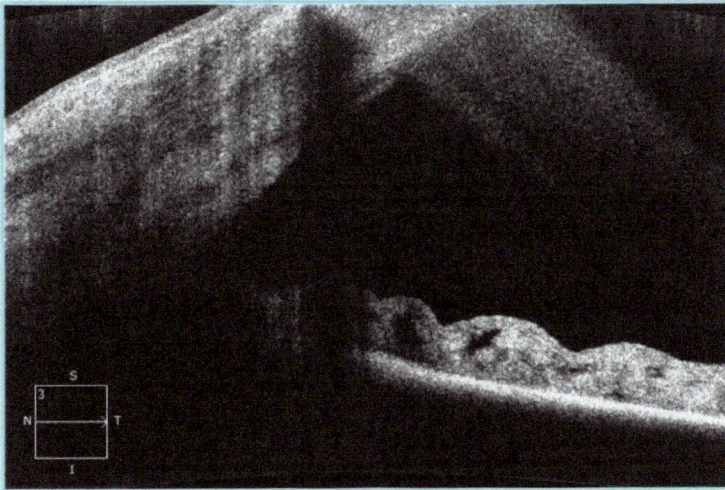

Fig. 4.23. Artefactual changes and inability to visualise iris insertion due to improper alignment.

of iris entry can sometimes be difficult to visualise due to a shadowing effect from the structures anterior to it.

Ultrasound Biomicroscopy (UBM)

UBM uses a high frequency ultrasound probe that is immersed in a water bath to give a detailed image of the anterior segment. A probe produces a soundwave of frequency of around 50MHz or higher. These soundwaves are reflected back to the probe head having passed to the tissue of interest to generate an electrical signal that can then produce the image seen.

Performing an ultrasound scan does require skill and experience to obtain satisfactory images. A detailed account of all the structures and lesions that can be found on ultrasound is beyond the scope of this book. The benefit of ultrasonography over OCT is that not only can the angle be assessed, but pathology affecting the iris or ciliary body that may be responsible for producing angle closure can be identified. For example, patients taking topiramate (an antiepileptic drug) can develop effusions that result in ciliary body oedema. The swollen ciliary body pushes

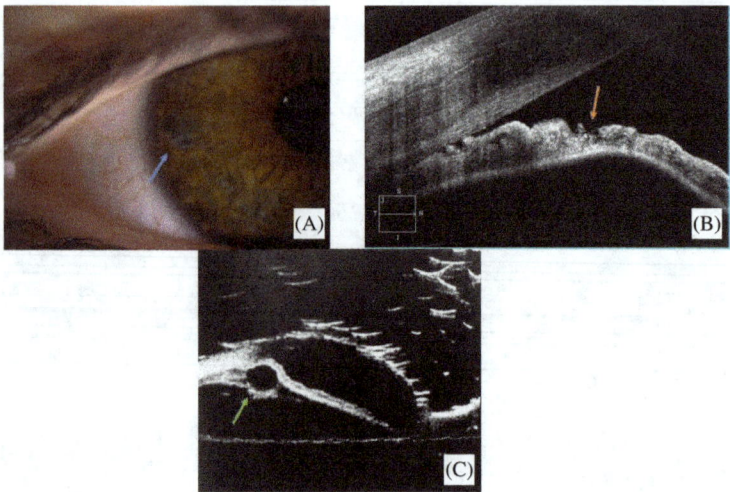

Fig. 4.24. Image A shows clinical suspicion of elevation of the iris (blue arrow). In Image B, OCT of the anterior segment confirms forward bowing of the iris but is unable to visualise the structures behind it (orange arrow). Image C shows a UBM image demonstrating a ciliary body cyst (green arrow).

anteriorly to result in a closed angle, usually bilaterally. UBM is a very useful tool for visualising these changes, which may affect further management. For example, peripheral iridotomy is highly unlikely to provide an effective solution to narrow angles caused by ciliary body pathology.

The drawback of using UBM is that it is operator dependant and requires experience to create reproducible images capable of being used to quantify angle measurements. The detail of the UBM scan is perhaps not as fine as the 5-line raster OCT. However, it is still possible to identify the scleral spur to grade the angle.

5

EYE DROPS

Andrew Swampillai

The mainstay treatment of chronic open angle and chronic angle closure glaucomas is medical therapy, with topical medications being the most common. All medications aim to reduce intraocular pressure by two main methods — either by decreasing aqueous humour production via action on the ciliary body or by facilitating outflow via the uveoscleral route.

Medical therapy may be in the form of

- aqueous drops (no blurring of vision but reduced contact time);
- gel suspension (slight blurring of vision but prolonged contact time);
- oral acetazolamide (prolonged effect on the eye but accompanied systemic side effects).

Only around 10% of most topical agents are absorbed into the eye. Absorption is dependent on a variety of factors including ocular contact time, drug concentration and tissue permeability. Small lipophilic drugs pass through the cornea, whereas larger hydrophilic drugs are generally absorbed through conjunctiva and sclera.

As there is no cure for glaucoma, a patient remains on some form of medical therapy for life in order to preserve their vision.

They may also remain on this even after undergoing laser treatment e.g. laser trabeculoplasty or cyclodiode. A patient will only stop using anti-glaucoma medication, if they undergo a form of glaucoma surgery, i.e. trabeculectomy or drainage tube insertion and the outcome is deemed successful.

APPLICATION TECHNIQUE

It is important to check with patients for correct application technique, so as to maximise the benefit of medical therapy in a lifetime. Incorrect application will eventually lead to inadequate intraocular pressure control and worsening of glaucoma. The way a patient can be taught to instil topical medication is as follows:

1. Wash hands before handling medication.
2. Pull lower eyelid down with the index and middle fingers of non-dominant hand.
3. With dominant hand, tilt bottle tip downwards and bring towards eye.
4. Invert bottle and squeeze to instil a single drop into the fornix created by pulling lower eyelid down — DO NOT TOUCH YOUR EYE OR EYELID WITH THE DROPPER TIP.
5. Close eye immediately and press on lacrimal sac area firmly for 1–2 minutes. This reduces systemic absorption and helps decrease systemic side effects.
6. Repeat in the other eye (if required).

Hints and tips:

- *If self-administration is unreliable, ensure that there is somebody (partner/relative/district nurse) who can assist them.*
- *Consider ways of making administering medication easier, e.g. lying flat on bed, mirror positioning, or eye drop dispensers. Smaller bottles and single-use vials can be particularly difficult to use in the frail and elderly.*
- *Aim to leave at least 5 minutes between instilling topical medication between both eyes.*

- *Space drops throughout the day and develop a regime to get into habit of administering, e.g. instilling drops before brushing teeth or before going to bed.*

TOPICAL ANTI-GLAUCOMA MEDICATION

Summarised below are a list of common anti-glaucoma drops and suspensions that are used in the United Kingdom.

Generic	Concentration	Dosage	Brand	Preservative Free
	Sympathomimetics (alpha agonists)			
Apraclonidine	0.5% 1%	TDS < 1month Pre-post anterior segment laser (YAG/ SLT)	Iopidine® 0.5%	Iopidine ® 1% single dose
Brimonidine tartrate	0.2%	BD	Alphagan®	n/a
	Carbonic Anhydrase Inhibitors			
Dorzolamide	2%	BD	Trusopt®	Trusopt® unit dose
Brinzolamide	1%	BD	Azopt®	n/a
	β-Blockers			
Betaxolol hydrochloride	0.25% 0.50%	BD BD	Betoptic ®suspension	Betoptic® suspension single dose 0.25%
Levobunlol hydrochloride	0.50%	BD	Betagan®	Betagan® unit dose
Timolol maleate	0.25% Gel 0.1%	BD OD	Timoptol® Tiopex®	Timpotol unit dose Tiopex®

Prostaglandin Analogues				
Latanoprost	0.005%	ON	Xalatan®	Monopost®
Bimatoprost	0.01%	ON	Lumigan®	
	0.03%	ON	0.01%	Lumigan® unit dose 0.03%
Travoprost	0.004%	ON	Travatan®	n/a
Tafluprost	0.0015%	ON		Saflutan® unit dose
Miotics				
Pilocarpine	1, 2 and 4%	TDS or QDS	Pilocarpine®	Minims (2%)® Pilocarpine nitrate
Combination Drops				
Latanoprost + Timolol	Latanoprost 0.005% + timolol 0.5%	ON	Xalacom® and others	Fixapost
Bimatoprost + Timolol	Bimatoprost 0.03% + timolol 0.5%	ON	Ganfort®	Ganfort® unit dose 0.03%
Travoprost + Timolol	Travaprost 0.004% + timolol 0.5%	ON	DuoTrav®	n/a
Brimonidine + Timolol	Brimonidine 0.2% + timolol 0.5%	BD	Combigan®	n/a
Brinzolamide + Timolol	Brinzolamide 1% + timolol 0.5%	BD	Azarga®	n/a
Dorzolamide + Timolol	Dorzolamide 2% + Timolol 0.5%	BD	Cosopt® and others	Cosopt® unit dose and others
Brinzolamide + Brimonidine	Brinzolamide 1% + Brimonidine 0.2%	BD	Simbrinza®	n/a

Abbreviations: *OD — once a day, BD — twice a day, TDS — three times a day, ON — at night*

It is important to check for any allergies and contraindications before drops are prescribed. **Non-selective β-blocker eye drops are contraindicated in patients with known asthma and chronic obstructive pulmonary disease.** Betaxolol is relatively safer than a non-selective β-blocker in patients with known reactive airway disease. However, the efficacy of betaxolol, despite being a relatively selective β-1-blocker, is less than that of non-selective β-blockers. **All β-blockers should be avoided in patients with bradycardia, heart block or heart failure.** Brimonidine eye drops should not be used in children aged below 12 years and are contraindicated in neonates and infants (less than 2 years of age). Consider preservative free preparations in very young patients, e.g. congenital or juvenile glaucoma or in those who have undergone previous corneal transplant surgery.

COMPLIANCE

Checking that patients take their medication is an essential part of ophthalmic care. It is estimated that up to 25–30% of patients may not be compliant with anti-glaucoma medication to varying degrees.

It is therefore worth inquiring as to why a patient may be non-compliant, e.g. side effects from drops, difficulty administering them, unaware of the importance of adherence to regimen, etc.

Compliance is also demonstrated to be more likely affected, if more than one anti-glaucoma medication is prescribed. This is worth bearing in mind, when reviewing a patient taking multiple drops. Practitioners should also suspect non-compliance if intraocular pressures are uncontrolled and there is evidence of visual field defect progression, although this should be approached with sensitivity.

Emphasis on developing a habit is important and can aide greatly i.e. routinely applying medication before brushing teeth or before going to sleep.

OCULAR SURFACE DISEASE

A considerable number of patients will eventually develop ocular surface disease, after many years of taking anti-glaucoma drops. This is mainly due to toxicity from drop preservatives (benzylkonium chloride) which are responsible for cell death in the corneal and conjunctival epithelium.

Ocular surface disease can lead to compliance issues and an adverse effect on any subsequent glaucoma surgery undertaken. Clinical signs of ocular surface disease include increasing conjunctival injection, persistent epithelial erosions and reduced tear film break-up. Consider switching such patients to preservative free medications where possible.

ANTI-GLAUCOMA MEDICATION IN PREGNANCY

The treatment of glaucoma in and around pregnancy offers a unique challenge of balancing the risk of vision loss to the mother against the potential harm to the foetus or newborn.

Brimonidine is generally the preferred first-line drug in the first, second and early third trimester. Late in the third trimester, Brimonidine should be discontinued because it can induce central nervous system depression in newborns, wherein topical Carbonic Anhydrase Inhibitors may be the optimal choice.

Prostaglandin analogues have been associated with a notable incidence of miscarriage in animal studies. They can increase uterine tone and stimulate uterine contractions producing premature labour. Since they may act as abortifacients, there are concerns regarding their use in pregnancy and are generally avoided.

Laser trabeculoplasty may be used as an adjunct or alternative to topical therapy in all trimesters.

COMMON SIDE EFFECTS

Class of Medication	Side Effects
PROSTAGLANDIN ANALOGUES	Increase in number of lashes
	Increased pigmentation of iris
	Uveitis
	Cystoid Macular Oedema
	Conjunctival Hyperemia
	Prostaglandin Associated Peri-orbitopathy
BETA BLOCKERS	Bradycardia
	Heart Block
	Bronchospasm
	Low Blood Pressure
	Decreased Libido
	CNS Depression
	B-1 selective-blockers like betaxolol have less pulmonary side effects
CARBONIC ANHYDRASE INHIBITORS	Metallic taste in mouth
	Oral Acetazolamide:
	Dehydration
	Hypokalemia
	Renal Stones
	Parasthesias
	DO NOT USE IF HISTORY OF SULFA ALLERGY (COMMONLY DESCRIBED AS ALLERGIC TO SEPTRIN WHICH IS A COMBINATION OF TRIMETHOPRIM AND SULFAMETHOXAZOLE)
SYMPATHOMIMETICS	Conjunctival Hyperemia

6

LASERS

Adam Booth

The control of intraocular pressure (IOP) is a balance between the production of aqueous humour by the ciliary body and the outflow of aqueous humour through the trabecular meshwork.

Laser treatment can either increase the outflow or reduce the production of aqueous humour, so leading to a reduction in IOP. The main advantage of laser over surgical treatment is that incisions do not need to be made into the eye, thus avoiding the risk of intraocular infection. Laser is therefore usually a safer treatment. Other advantages are that it is quick, follow up is usually less and both eyes can be treated at the same time. It is therefore quite often preferred by patients to surgery.

INCREASE OUTFLOW

Selective Laser Trabeculoplasty (SLT)

The function of SLT is to reduce IOP by increasing the outflow of aqueous humour through the trabecular meshwork. It is suitable for patients with primary open angle glaucoma and some secondary glaucomas. The forerunner to SLT was Argon Laser Trabeculoplasty. This is now rarely performed.

SLT increases aqueous humour outflow by both releasing cytokines and also activating trabeculocyte cells which remove debris from the trabecular meshwork.

Patients are pre-treated with iopidine 1% drops to prevent a post laser rise in IOP. Patients may also be pre-treated with pilocarpine 2% drops to aid visualization of the trabecular meshwork. Topical anaesthetic drops are also instilled.

SLT is performed with a slit lamp mounted laser. SLT and YAG lasers are often combined into a single delivery system. It is therefore essential that the correct laser type is selected by the doctor. A contact gonioscopy lens is placed on the patient's eye to enable the trabecular meshwork to be visualised.

Laser shots are placed one burn width apart over the trabecular meshwork. The initial laser power used is 0.7mJ. The power can slowly be turned up until small bubbles are seen at which point the power is turned down by 0.1mJ. Up to 360° degrees of trabecular meshwork can be treated at one session. SLT takes about 5 minutes per eye. Both eyes can be treated at the same sitting. Patients can be aware of bright flashing lights during SLT but usually feel either no or only slight discomfort.

SLT has an 85–90% success rate in lowering IOP. The reduction in IOP can take 1 week to 1 month to occur. The effects of SLT last 2–4 years and then wear off. SLT can then be repeated with equal success.

SLT has little risks or side effects. It can cause a temporary rise in IOP soon after the treatment. The IOP should therefore be checked about an hour post laser. It often causes a mild transient anterior uveitis. Many doctors will therefore prescribe ketorolac (a non-steroidal anti-inflammatory agent) drops to be used three times a day for three days.

Patients should continue their glaucoma drops after SLT unless advised otherwise by their doctor. Patients can continue normal activity after laser with no restrictions. Follow up should be in 4–8 weeks to assess the initial effects of the laser.

TO OPEN THE DRAINAGE ANGLE

YAG Laser Peripheral Iridotomy

The aim of laser peripheral iridotomy (PI) is to open or widen a narrow or closed anterior chamber drainage angle. A small hole is made in the peripheral iris using a YAG laser. This may be performed either prophylactically to prevent acute angle closure glaucoma or to treat established acute angle closure glaucoma. It is also occasionally used to treat patients with forms of pupil block glaucoma.

Patients are pre-treated with pilocarpine 2% drops in order to constrict the pupil. This both thins the peripheral iris making it easier to make a hole in it and also prevents IOP rise post laser. Patients should be warned that the pilocarpine drops often cause a temporary frontal headache and dimming of the vision. Iopidine (apraclonidine) 1% drops are also usually used to prevent a rise in IOP post laser. Local anaesthetic drops are instilled. If a patient has acute glaucoma the IOP needs to be controlled before performing a PI.

YAG PI laser is performed with an iridotomy contact lens. Usually a single small hole in the iris is made. It can be placed either under the upper lid or at 3 or 9 o'clock. The power is usually set at 1.0 mJ initially and then slowly increased until a hole is formed in the peripheral iris. Patients often describe an unusual rather than a painful sensation during laser. Laser PI can take just a few seconds in a patient with a thin blue iris but can take a few minutes in a patient with a thick dark iris. Occasionally people with very thick irises can be pre-treated with Argon laser.

The side effects of YAG PI laser are usually minor. There are several small blood vessels on the iris which can bleed if hit with the laser shot. Bleeding can easily be stopped by pressing on the contact lens for a few seconds. It is important to check IOP about 30 minutes post laser to check for a transient rise. Patients are usually prescribed a topical steroid to be used 4 times a day for 1-week post laser to treat the mild anterior uveitis which can occur. Patients can occasionally complain of seeing a line of light in their inferior vision after YAG PI. This can be avoided by not performing the PI at the upper lid margin.

Patients should continue their pre-laser drops unless otherwise advised. Their vision can be blurred for the rest of the day but returns to normal by the next day. There are no restrictions to a patient's activity after laser.

Laser Peripheral Iridoplasty

Patients are reviewed approximately 1 month after YAG PI. If the drainage angle is still found to be narrow then laser peripheral iridoplasty can be performed. This involves making 12 gentle burns with the argon or similar laser to the peripheral iris. The burns cause slight shrinkage of the peripheral iris so pulling the iris out of the anterior drainage angle and therefore opening up the angle.

REDUCE INFLOW

Cyclodiode

Cyclodiode laser is used to partially destroy the ciliary body and so reduce the production of aqueous humour. It is usually used in patients with secondary glaucoma with a poor visual prognosis, e.g. rubeotic glaucoma. However, it can also be used in patients with primary glaucomas.

Patients undergoing cyclodiode laser require a local anaesthetic injection, ideally a peribulbar block. It is therefore usually performed in theatre with an anaesthetist present. Patients do not require drops prior to their laser treatment.

Before starting cyclodiode the position of the ciliary body is identified by retro illumination. Cyclodiode laser is then applied with a G-probe with the edge of the probe placed at the limbus. The power is initially set at 1500 mW with a duration of 1500 mS. This can be increased up to 2000 mW for 2000 mS. If one hears a pop, then the laser power should be turned down.

There is some variation in how many clock hours are treated per session. One suggested regime is to treat 270° per session. The 3 and 9 o'clock positions should be avoided in order to avoid the long ciliary nerves and minimize pain. Cyclodiode laser takes about 10 minutes. Sub-conjunctival steroid can be given at the end of the procedure to reduce inflammation.

Cyclodiode laser is highly effective at reducing IOP. If the initial treatment does not lower the pressure sufficiently then it can be repeated.

Inflammation is the main side effect of cyclodiode laser. Patients are treated with frequent topical steroids post laser to reduce the inflammation. Hypotony, with an IOP less than 6 mm Hg, can occasionally occur.

Endoscopic cyclodiode laser can also be performed, usually combined with phacoemulsification. The laser probe and camera are inserted into the anterior segment and lasering of the ciliary body takes place under direct visualization.

MISCELLANEOUS

Argon Suture Lysis

The argon, or similar laser, can be used to cut trabeculectomy flap sutures if drainage post trabeculectomy is found to be insufficient. This allows the scleral flap to open so increasing the flow of aqueous humour out of the eye. A Hoskins lens is usually used. The lens is pressed onto the conjunctiva over the suture which needs to be cut. This brings the suture into sharp focus so allowing the laser to cut the suture.

YAG Goniopuncture

If there is insufficient drainage of aqueous humour after non-penetrating glaucoma surgery such as deep sclerectomy or visco-canalostomy, then a YAG goniopuncture can be performed. The YAG laser is used to make a hole in Descemet's window, so increasing the outflow of aqueous humour and a reduction in IOP.

Pan-retinal Photocoagulation for Iris/Angle Neovascularisation

New vessels can grow on the iris or drainage angle after conditions such as proliferative diabetic retinopathy or retinal vascular occlusions. These new vessels can cause rubeotic glaucoma to develop. The mainstay of treatment is pan retinal photocoagulation where 2000–3000 burns are placed on the peripheral retina using the argon or similar laser. This results in regression of the new vessels.

7

SURGERY

Abhijit A Mohite and Imran Masood

Glaucoma surgery is traditionally offered to patients when eye drops and/or laser (selective laser trabeculoplasty) have failed to achieve target IOP levels or prevent progressive visual field loss.

Because of the infrequent but significant risks associated with traditional 'incisional' surgeries, surgery tends to be reserved for patients with definite evidence of glaucoma progression or with very high IOP despite maximum tolerated medical therapy.

Surgery is offered to some patients to achieve drop-independence, either because of inability to reliably instil drops or intolerable side effects from drops.

Hence, the indications for glaucoma surgery can be summarised as follows:

- Failure of medical or laser therapy to achieve adequate IOP control or stabilisation of disease progression.
- Avoidance of excessive polypharmacy in order to avoid side effects or ocular surface toxicity from chronic drop use.
- As primary therapy in advanced disease at presentation requiring a very low target IOP, particularly in younger patients.

- For patient preference if the patient has a strong preference to be drop-independent long term.
- Poor patient compliance with medical treatment.

With the introduction of a variety of Minimally Invasive Glaucoma Surgery (MIGS) procedures over the last decade, newer conjunctiva-sparing ('non-incisional') glaucoma surgeries are increasingly being offered earlier in the course of disease. Although IOP reduction with MIGS is usually less profound, their safer risk profile and ability to combine them with cataract surgery ('phaco-plus' procedures) has meant MIGS are increasingly being offered to patients who have early-to-moderate and/ or non-progressive disease.

This often means patients no longer need eye drops to achieve disease control, which effectively then eradicates the all-too-common problems of poor patient compliance and lack of adherence to drop regimes. The added benefit of drop independence is that the ocular surface is spared from the toxic, pro-inflammatory effects of many glaucoma drops which can compromise the success rates of any future incisional surgery that may be required.

INCISIONAL SURGERY

When the target IOP to achieve glaucoma control is low, filtration or incisional surgery remains the option of choice. Aside from potential complications, which are discussed later, these surgeries are fraught with the problems of the healing (or scarring) response which inevitably ensues. Scar formation by tenon's and conjunctival fibroblast cells can lead to subsequent surgical failure as outflow drainage is gradually impeded.

There are several well recognised ocular and patient factors that increase the risk of scarring after glaucoma filtration surgery (Table 7.1). Multiple risk factors confer additional risk of scarring, and therefore it is important to risk stratify patients in this regard when planning incisional surgery.

Table 7.1. Risk factors for scarring after glaucoma filtration (incisional) surgery.

Ocular	Patient
Previous conjunctival surgery — e.g. squint surgery, retinal detachment surgery	African-Caribbean origin — West African greater risk than East African
Chronic conjunctival inflammation	Indian Subcontinent origin
Previous failed filtration surgery	Hispanic origin
Previous cataract extraction — if conjunctival incision	Younger age (<40)
Aphakia	Children
Uveitis — active, persistent	
Neovascular glaucoma	
Long term topical medication use — especially if they cause a red eye	
Time since last surgery — especially if within last 30 days	
Other secondary glaucomas — e.g. iridocorneal endothelial syndrome, post-traumatic angle recession	

Antimetabolites and Glaucoma Surgery

To prevent failure due to scarring, antimetabolites are now routinely used to modulate the healing response and 'augment' such procedures through their anti-fibrotic effects. The most commonly used are **mitomycin C** (MMC) and **5-fluorouracil** (5-FU), which were both introduced in the 1980's as adjuncts to trabeculectomy and act to inhibit fibroblast proliferation and activity. MMC is an alkylating agent that inhibits multiplication of the fibroblast cells that produce scar tissue by cross-linking their DNA, whereas 5-FU reduces fibroblast activity by blocking DNA synthesis and is a less aggressive antimetabolite. Because of their strong cytotoxic effects, both are associated with some complications which are often dose dependant (Table 7.2), and

Table 7.2. Potential complications of antimetabolites.

Chronic hypotony (defined as IOP below 6 mm Hg with worsening of vision)

Wound edge leaks

Limbal stem cell failure

Epithelial erosions — mainly with 5-FU subconjunctival injections

Intraocular penetration and damage — including endothelial loss and ciliary body destruction

Infection — blebitis and endophthalmitis due to cystic thin-walled blebs

Scleral thinning and necrosis

Malignancy/teratogenicity — avoid use if patient is pregnant

therefore their intra-operative use requires meticulous care and surgical technique.

Incisional glaucoma surgery can broadly be divided into *penetrating* and *non-penetrating* procedures, depending on whether the anterior chamber (AC) is directly entered or not. The principal penetrating surgeries are trabeculectomy and tube shunts (also known as glaucoma drainage implants).

Penetrating Glaucoma Filtration Surgery

• Trabeculectomy

Widely regarded as the gold-standard glaucoma operation, the trabeculectomy has been around since the 1960's. It creates a fistula between the AC and the anterior subconjunctival space through which aqueous can drain, and begins by making a 4–6 mm circumferential conjunctival incision at the limbus (peritomy) to create a fornix-based conjunctival flap (Fig. 7.1A). Next, MMC is applied onto the scleral bed for 1–3 minutes and irrigated with balanced salt solution (BSS). A rectangular scleral flap of half-thickness depth is then fashioned (Fig. 7.1B), before releasable sutures are pre-placed (commonly two, one at each flap corner) prior to entering the AC. At this stage a temporal corneal paracentesis is created. An AC maintainer, which feeds

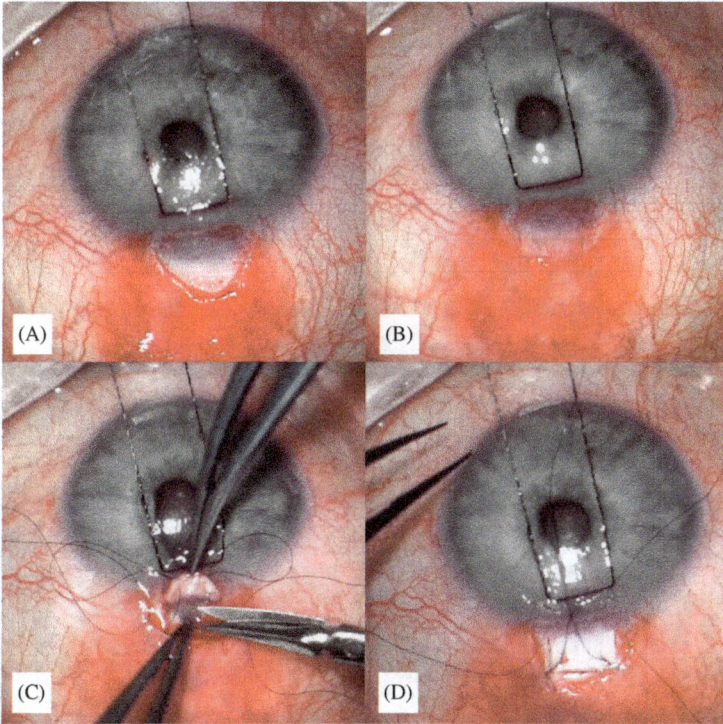

Fig. 7.1. Trabeculectomy.

BSS into the eye via a three-way tap, is sometimes also inserted at this stage to prevent shallowing of the chamber when entered. The anterior chamber is then entered using a surgical blade, and a small sclerotomy and peripheral iridectomy (excision of scleral and iris tissue, respectively) are created (Fig. 7.1C). The former creates an adequately-sized aqueous outflow pathway, whilst the latter prevents the peripheral iris from becoming incarcerated in the newly created scleral opening. Despite its name, modern trabeculectomy is no longer performed as an excision of the relatively posterior trabecular meshwork. Instead, the AC is entered more anteriorly with excision of the posterior cornea and anterior sclera, as this reduces the risk of ciliary body bleeding as well as iris incarceration.

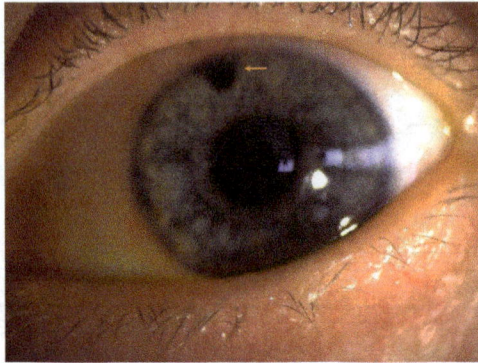

Fig. 7.2. Appearance of surgical iridectomy done as part of a trabeculectomy procedure (orange arrow).

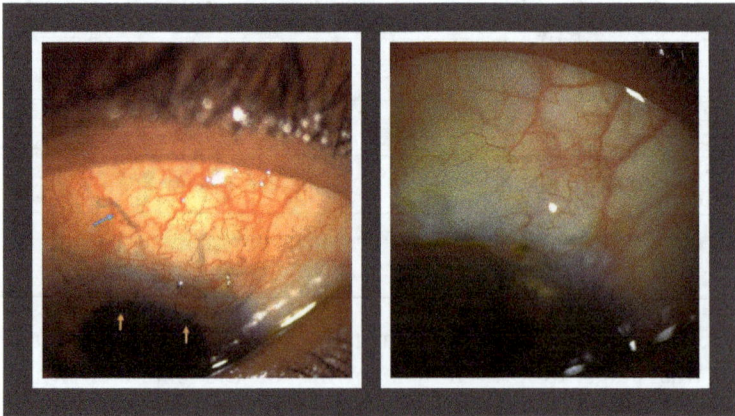

Fig. 7.3. Appearance of a bleb one day after trabeculectomy (left image). The bleb is mostly flat, with conjunctival congestion. The distal end of one of the releasable sutures is visible under the conjunctiva (blue arrow). The orange arrows show proximal corneal loops of the releasable sutures. Pulling on these loops causes the distal knot to come undone, thereby allowing removal of the suture and enhanced drainage from the scleral flap. The same bleb six months later (right image). A diffuse bleb can be seen with no conjunctival congestion. In this case both releasable sutures have been subsequently removed.

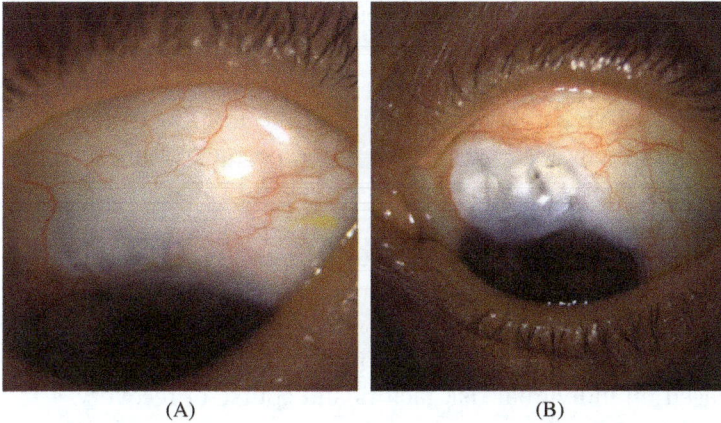

(A)   (B)

Fig. 7.4. Different types of blebs. Figure (A) shows a diffuse bleb. Figure (B) shows a more localised, anteriorly placed and thin walled bleb.

The scleral flap is then secured tightly by tying the pre-placed releasable sutures to allow some minimal drainage (Fig. 7.1D), before the conjunctiva is finally sutured back to the limbus to ensure water-tight closure.

Complications

Trabeculectomy demands exacting surgical technique as each step is critical in ensuring a good surgical outcome. Close review in the post-operative period is crucial in ensuring the success of the procedure, so that problems such as over-filtration, under-filtration and excessive scarring can be detected and managed as early as possible.

Post-Operative

Post-operative drop regimes can vary from surgeon to surgeon but mostly involve

— cessation of all glaucoma drops in operated eye;
— steroid eye drops (preferably preservative free) such as Dexamethasone 0.1% 2 hourly during waking hours for three months;

— a steroid ointment such as Betnesol at night for three months;
— an antibiotic eye drop such as Chloramphenicol four times
a day for two weeks;
— a parasympatholytic eye drop in the form of Atropine 1%
once a day for a week (this prevents aqueous misdirection,
particularly in phakic eyes).

Post-operative follow-up is usually at Day 1, Week 1, Week
2, Week 4, Week 8, Week 12 and then at 4 months. After this
the patient usually reverts back to 6 monthly glaucoma follow
ups. However, the follow up intervals can be very variable
based on individual risk factors and course of recovery.

Table 7.3 summarises the main post-operative complications.

Recent innovations have sought to augment existing trabeculectomy techniques with devices to reduce associated risks
of over-drainage and hypotony. These include the Ex-PRESS

Table 7.3. Post-operative complications after trabeculectomy.

Over-filtration	o Large bleb, shallow AC, low IOP <6 mmHg o Hypotony-choroidal detachment o Hypotonous maculopathy
Under-filtration	o Shallow bleb, deep AC, high IOP
Bleb leakage	—
Hyphema	—
Inflammation	o Ciliary body shutdown and subsequent hypotony
Iris incarceration into sclerotomy	o Incomplete peripheral iridectomy
Aqueous misdirection	o Variable bleb, shallow AC, high IOP
Suprachoroidal haemorrhage	o Variable bleb, shallow AC, variable IOP
Early and late bleb failure	—
Visual 'wipe out' in advanced glaucoma	—
Early and late bleb related infections	o Blebitis o Endophthalmitis

shunt, which is inserted into the AC during trabeculectomy instead of creating a sclerectomy and iridectomy.

- **Glaucoma Drainage Implants (tube shunts)**

Whilst trabeculectomy filters aqueous into the anterior sub-conjunctival space, more posterior filtration behind the equator reduces the extent of the post-operative fibrotic response by means of it being further away from the 'active' limbal zone. Glaucoma drainage implants (GDIs) work on this notion by shunting aqueous from the AC via a silicone tube to a plate fixated to the post-equatorial sclera. The plate causes a fibrotic response within the tenons layer which gradually encloses it with a thin capsule of connective tissue over a period of 2–3 weeks. When aqueous drains into the plate from the AC, it distends this capsule to form a single chamber sub-conjunctival reservoir ('bleb') which is in free communication with the AC.

There are two principle types of GDI — *valved* and *non-valved*. Valved implants provide resistance to aqueous flow from the outset, thereby preventing hypotony in the early post-operative period. Non-valved implants provide no resistance to flow until the fibrous capsule forms around the episcleral plate. They therefore require occluding via internal stent sutures (placed within the lumen) and external dissolvable ligation sutures to limit early flow and prevent early hypotony. The tube is usually covered with a patch graft of donor sclera or specially processed pericardium ('Tutoplast') to prevent erosion through the overlying conjunctiva. For non-valved implants venting slit are often created in the tube in front of the ligation suture to allow some early flow in eyes where some immediate IOP lowering is required. It must be remembered that for non-valved implants, patients will require a second operation to remove the internal stent suture thereby allowing the procedure to show its full IOP lowering effect. This is usually done 2–3 months after the initial procedure (allowing time for conjunctival fibrosis to develop beyond the plate margin, thereby ensuring the filtration bleb is formed only above the plate itself). This prevents over-filtration and hypotony.

GDI's are usually indicated when there is extensive conjunctival scarring, a previous trabeculectomy has failed, or there is a high risk of trabeculectomy failure due to scarring. As discussed earlier, these include neovascular glaucoma, uveitic glaucoma, glaucoma associated with corneal grafts, irido-corneal endothelial syndrome, paediatric glaucoma, and glaucoma following retinal detachment surgery (Table 7.1).

Baerveldt Tube

This non-valved device is available in three sizes of episcleral plates — 250 mm^2, 350 mm^2 and 500 mm^2. The plate's fenestrations allow fibrous tissue to grow through them, thereby reducing the height of the bleb and reducing the risk of post-operative diplopia. The wings of the plate have to be positioned underneath two rectus muscles.

Ahmed Valve

This is a valved device which consists of two thin silicone elastic membranes positioned in a venture-shaped chamber. The elastic membranes restrict flow up to a pressure of 8–12 mmHg. The device plate is available in a variety of sizes and also comes in single and double-plated versions. It is placed in between rectus muscles.

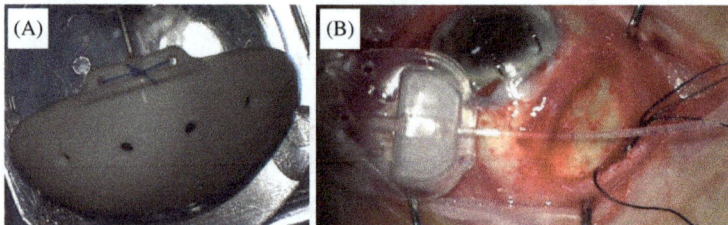

Fig. 7.5. Two types of Glaucoma drainage implants — Baerveldt (A) and Ahmed (B).

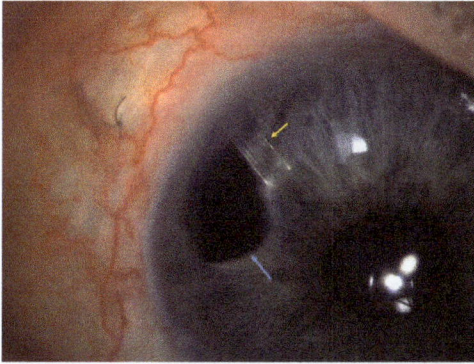

Fig. 7.6. Ahmed Valve tube seen in position in the anterior chamber (yellow arrow). The Baerveldt tube would also present with a similar appearance in the anterior chamber. This patient has an area of iris trauma from a previous ocular injury (blue arrow).

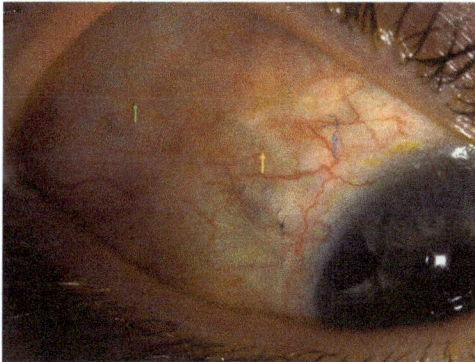

Fig. 7.7. Patient with Ahmed Valve. Image shows sutures used to secure the pericardial patch (blue arrow), the tube under the pericardial patch/conjunctiva (yellow arrow) and a bleb over the episcleral plate (green arrow).

Molteno Tube

This is a non-valved implant which is available in single and double-plated versions and is also placed in between rectus muscles. Each plate has a 13 mm diameter and a surface area of 134 mm^2. A smaller plate size is also available for paediatric eyes.

Complications:

Table 7.4. Post-operative complications after Glaucoma Drainage Implants (GDIs)

	Notes
Over-filtration	o Large bleb, shallow AC, low IOP o Hypotony — choroidal detachment o Hypotony maculopathy
Under-filtration	o Blockage of tube by iris, fibrin, blood or vitreous
Hyphema	o From iris trauma during AC entry
Inflammation	o Ciliary body shutdown and subsequent hypotony
Corneal decompensation	o Malposition of tube closer to endothelium
Tube retraction and erosion	o Exposure can lead to endophthalmitis
Tube kinking	o Causes tube obstruction
Late bleb encapsulation	o Excessive thickening of the plate capsule
Diplopia	—
Visual 'wipe out' in advanced glaucoma	—
Suprachoroidal haemorrhage	—
Retinal detachment	—

Post-operative

Post-operative drops usually involve:

— cessation of glaucoma drops in operated eye;
— antibiotic eye drops for four weeks (such as Chloramphenicol four times a day);
— steroid eye drops (such as Dexamethasone 0.1%) four times a day for six weeks.

Post-operative follow-up is usually at Day 1, Week 1, Week 3, Week 6 and at 3 months, following which patient reverts to usual glaucoma follow-up schedule. However, both the post-operative drops and follow-up schedule can vary on a case by case basis and will be determined by the supervising clinician.

- **Preserflo Microshunt**

This is a newer and smaller non-valved tube shunt that is not yet widely used in the UK, although it has been approved in Europe since 2012. The tube is made of a stable, highly biocompatible synthetic polymer and measures 8.5 mm in length, has a small 70 μm lumen diameter and a 1.1 mm width fin located halfway along its length to help secure it within the sclera. The device has no plate and instead is designed to shunt aqueous into the anterior subconjunctival space much like a trabeculectomy. Surgery involves very similar dissection to a trabeculectomy including a limbal peritomy, application of MMC onto the scleral bed, and conjunctival closure. However, rather than creating a scleral flap, sclerotomy and iridectomy, a needle is advanced through a scleral pocket to enter the AC through the irido-corneal angle. Early results are promising, but as this device relies on anterior subconjunctival filtration, it is faced with the same perils of subconjunctival fibrosis and failure as trabeculectomy surgery but with lower risk of hypotony due to its narrow lumen diameter.

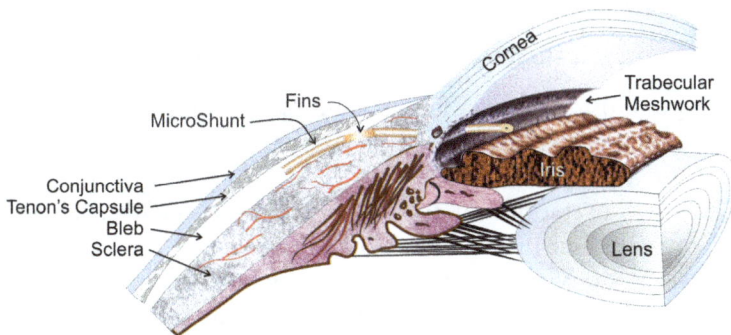

Fig. 7.8. Preserflo microshunt (Image courtesy of Santen Pharmaceutical Co Ltd).

Non-penetrating Glaucoma Filtration Surgery

• Deep Sclerectomy

This is an incisional surgery where the anterior chamber is not penetrated; no full thickness opening is created like in a trabeculectomy. Instead a superficial scleral flap is fashioned, a second deeper scleral flap of 90% thickness is excised and then the Schlemm's Canal (SC) is de-roofed to expose only the SC (and TM beneath). This allows aqueous to seep through a thin semipermeable membrane of tissue into the newly created scleral lake and onwards into the subconjunctival space via the superficial flap. A collage implant is sometimes placed to maintain the scleral lake, before the superficial flap and conjunctiva are closed.

Deep sclerectomy is technically extremely challenging but confers lower risks of hypotony and over-filtration since drainage occurs across semi-permeable ocular structures that act as a barrier and provide some outflow resistance. As the AC is not penetrated, intraocular infection, inflammation, cataract formation and bleeding risks are also lower. However, given the steep learning curve and longer duration of the surgery it is not commonly performed across the UK. Inadvertent perforation of the Descemet membrane during deep flap dissection and entry into the AC is not uncommon even in experienced hands, essentially then converting the procedure into a trabeculectomy.

• Viscocanalostomy/Canaloplasty/Trabeculotomy

Viscocanalostomy is a non-penetrating filtering surgery very similar to deep sclerectomy (DS). A superficial scleral flap, excision of a deep scleral flap and de-roofing of the Schlemm's Canal are performed in the same way. A specially designed cannula is then introduced into the cut end of the SC and a high-viscosity viscoelastic device is injected into it to dilate the canal and improve physiological outflow via the conventional pathway. The superficial flap and conjunctiva are then closed as before.

Canaloplasty is a variation of this procedure, whereby a fibre optic illuminated microcatheter ('iTrack') is used to circumferentially cannulate the entire 360° of the SC prior to injection of viscoelastic through the catheter to dilate the canal.

Trabeculotomy is a similar non-penetrating procedure that involves making the same initial deep dissection as DS and viscocanalostomy. It was first described for the treatment of primary congenital glaucoma in children. A fibre optic micro-catheter or Prolene suture is used to circumferentially cannu-late the SC in exactly the same way as for a canaloplasty. However, rather than dilate the SC with viscoelastic the micro-catheter or suture is then pulled through the canal into the anterior chamber so that the TM is cleaved, leaving the aque-ous in direct communication with the SC and collector channels of the distal outflow system.

NON-INCISIONAL SURGERY

Minimally invasive glaucoma surgery (MIGS) procedures form a heterogenous group of conjunctiva-sparing techniques that can

- bypass the Trabecular Meshwork (TM);
- excise the TM;
- dilate the canal of Schlemm;
- shunt aqueous into the suprachoroidal space;
- shunt aqueous into the subconjunctival space;
- reduce aqueous production from the ciliary body.

MIGS is a term that has become widely adopted to encom-pass a range of non-incisional glaucoma procedures with the following characteristics that distinguish it from traditional incisional glaucoma surgery:

- Minimal or no surgical manipulation of the conjunctiva and sclera. MIGS procedures therefore should not preclude the possibility or limit the success of future incisional surgeries such as trabeculectomy or tube shunts.
- The devices or procedures are usually approached from inside the eye (*ab interno*) via a clear corneal incision, and often require a surgical gonioscope for visualisation.

- More modest IOP lowering effects compared to trabeculectomy but can effectively reduce dependence on topical medications.
- Higher safety profile.
- More rapid visual recovery requiring few, if any, post-operative manipulations.
- Can often be combined with phacoemulsification surgery in eyes with both cataract and glaucoma.

Numerous videos of the various methods are available on YouTube.

Trabecular Bypass

If the drainage angle is open (no irido-trabecular contact) then outflow impedance is thought to be principally at the level of the TM, with the greatest resistance in open-angle glaucoma thought to be at the juxtacanalicular TM and the adjacent inner wall of the Schlemm's Canal. This is especially true in secondary open-angle glaucomas such as pseudo-exfoliation, pigment dispersion and steroid-induced glaucoma. Aqueous has to traverse through the TM before entering the distal outflow pathways of the SC and the collector channels. Therefore, either bypassing the TM with stents to access the SC or excising the TM to expose the inner wall of the SC should reduce resistance and lower IOP by increasing aqueous flow via the conventional physiological outflow pathway.

There are several trabecular microbypass devices in current practice, the most common of which are the iStent, iStent inject and Hydrus devices. All are inserted into the drainage angle *ab interno* under gonioscopic guidance via a temporal clear corneal incision and act as stents draining aqueous from the AC directly into the SC by bypassing the diseased TM. All are commonly inserted as stand-alone procedures or at the end of cataract surgery in patients with combined cataracts and glaucoma.

- **iStent/iStent Inject**

The iStent is a first-generation titanium trans-trabecular stent that was first introduced in 2007. It is 1mm long, 250 μm wide,

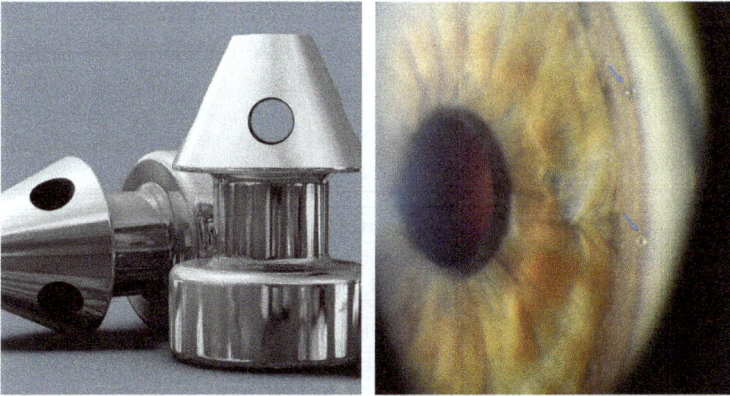

Fig. 7.9. iStent inject animation (image on left), and as seen on goni-oscopy after successful implantation (blue arrows in image on right). Image courtesy of Glaukos Corporation.

heparin-coated, has a snorkel shape and sits within the SC. It has a self-trephining angled tip and is manually inserted through the TM. Several studies have shown that combined iStent with phacoemulsification surgery significantly outper-forms phacoemulsification alone in terms of both IOP reduction and long-term topical anti-glaucoma medication use.

The iStent inject is the second-generation of the iStent and is a smaller version of the original model, with a completely different design. It consists of two 360 μm long and 230 μm wide, heparin-coated bolt shaped titanium stents pre-loaded into an auto-injector that allows implantation through the TM via a click-and-release motion.

- **Hydrus Microstent**

This 8 mm long curved stent is made of nitinol (highly biocom-patible material used in cardiovascular stents) and curved to match the curvature of the SC. It's designed to sit within the SC and has three 'windows' that face the anterior chamber and acts to both scaffold open around 3 clock hours of the SC and bypass the TM. A recent multi-centre randomised trial has demonstrated lower IOPs at two years after combined phacoemulsification and

Hydrus surgery compared to phacoemulsification alone. The Hydrus microstent has recently been FDA-approved but is not commonly used in the UK as yet.

Trabecular Excision

Other MIGS procedures enhance physiological outflow by removing either an arc or all 360° of TM and its adjacent inner wall of the SC. This permits aqueous direct access to the SC and the collector channels of the distal outflow system. Again, these procedures are performed either combined with phacoemulsification surgery or as stand-alone surgery.

- **Trabectome**

Available since 2006, this device is essentially a microscopic electrocautery instrument with a special tip that removes approximately a 15- to 30-degree arc of the TM and the SC inner wall tissue with an electro-surgical ablative pulse. The Trabectome is inserted *ab interno* through a clear corneal incision and is advanced either clockwise or counterclockwise through the anterior chamber angle under direct gonioscopic visualisation.

- **Kahook Dual Blade**

Like the Trabectome, this technique allows for localised excision of the TM and inner wall of the SC. Rather than electro-cautery, the Kahook dual blade is a specially designed blade that causes no thermal damage to surrounding tissues.

- **Gonioscopy-Assisted-Transluminal-Trabeculotomy (GATT)**

The GATT procedure is a newer *ab interno* circumferential trabeculotomy that works very much on the same principles of the incisional non-penetrating (*ab externo*) trabeculotomy described earlier, but with the added benefits of being a MIGS procedure.

Through a temporal clear corneal incision and under gonioscopic view, a blade is used to incise the TM over 2 clock hours (a goniotomy) to expose the SC. Either a blunted Prolene suture or lighted fibre-optic microcatheter (iTrack, Ellex) in introduced into the AC through a separate corneal incision and then guided through the goniotomy into the SC using microsurgical forceps introduced via the temporal corneal incision. The catheter is advanced circumferentially until 360° cannulation of the SC is achieved, and the tip comes out of the opposite side of the goniotomy. Whilst the internal leading end of the catheter is grasped with the microsurgical forceps, the external end is gradually pulled out through the second corneal incision to cause cleavage of the entire TM and complete the trabeculotomy.

Disadvantages of the procedure include the need for a clear cornea and the common post-operative complication of a transient hyphema due to episcleral venous backflow.

Schlemm's Canal Dilation

MIGS procedures that dilate the Schlemm's Canal *ab interno* work in the same principal as non-penetrating incisional procedures such as viscocanalostomy and canaloplasty, in that they circumferentially dilate the SC to create multiple micro-ruptures of the inner and outer SC endothelial lining. This is thought to reduce resistance, enhance physiological outflow and therefore reduce IOP.

Schlemm's Canal procedures have the advantage of low hypotony risk (IOP <6 mmHg) because the distal outflow pathway beyond the SC has a physiological IOP floor of around 10 mmHg; attributed to the episcleral venous pressure (EVP). Because these procedures cannot reduce outflow resistance distal to the SC, such as the episcleral veins, they should not be used in patients requiring low IOP targets below episcleral venous pressure. Examples include patients with scleral buckles, Grave's disease, or Sturge-Weber syndrome, all of which are conditions with raised EVP. They are best reserved for patients with normal EVP and baseline IOP higher than EVP. The same principle also applies to all the other described MIGS procedures, except those that target the subconjunctival space or decrease production of aqueous by the ciliary body.

- **Ab interno Canaloplasty (ABiC)**

ABiC is a new technique that draws on the same principles as external canaloplasty, described earlier, but with the benefits of being a MIGS procedure. This surgery is very similar to the GATT procedure, whereby a lighted fibre-optic microcatheter is introduced circumferentially into the SC under gonioscopic visualisation. However, rather than cleave the catheter out through the TM and into the AC, small aliquots of viscoelastic are injected through it to dilate the SC as the catheter is carefully withdrawn back out in the opposite direction.

Suprachoroidal Space

Up to 50% of normal aqueous outflow from the eye is via the uveoscleral pathway. Of note, the most effective topical hypotensive medication, the prostaglandin analogues, exert their effect via this pathway. Targeting this physiological pathway by stenting open the suprachoroidal space is therefore another interesting option in the glaucoma surgical armamentarium.

- **Cypass Microstent**

This stent is 6.35 mm long slightly curved polyamide tube that is 510 μm wide and has retention rings located at the anterior chamber end to help anchor it. It has fenestrations along its length designed to improve filtration into the suprachoroidal space and is inserted on a guidewire through a clear corneal incision under gonioscopic visualisation. The tip of the guidewire is used to dissect the ciliary body from the scleral spur, before the stent is advanced into the suprachoroidal space.

It was withdrawn voluntarily by its manufacturer (Alcon) in August 2018, because of concerns over increased loss of endothelial cells in some patients over 5 years of follow-up.

- **iStent Supra**

Due to be commercially available soon, the iStent Supra is inserted in a similar fashion to the Cypass. It is a more curved 4 mm long heparin-coated tube made of polyethersulfone and titanium with a 165 μm lumen diameter and no fenestrations.

Subconjunctival Space

Shunting of aqueous into the subconjunctival space without creating a window in the scleral wall (as in a trabeculectomy) can be achieved by stenting the TM and sclera via an *ab interno* approach. These procedures bypass physiological outflow pathways entirely and create filtering subconjunctival blebs, like trabeculectomy blebs, which require similar bleb monitoring and management of subconjunctival-episcleral fibrosis.

• Xen Gel Stent

This is a 6 mm long soft collage-derived porcine gelatin stent that is pre-loaded into an injector device so that it can be implanted *ab interno* to create a drainage pathway from the anterior chamber directly into the anterior subconjunctival space. It is often augmented with mitomycin C to prevent episcleral fibrosis. The stent comes in different lumen diameters — 45 μm, 63 μm or 140 μm — although the risk of over-drainage and hypotony is increased with the larger diameter stents.

Reducing Production of Aqueous by the Ciliary Body

All the MIGS procedures described above aim to improve aqueous outflow by bypassing or enhancing the physiological aqueous outflow pathways that are known to be diseased in eyes with glaucoma. Cyclodestructive procedures, however, lower IOP by reducing aqueous production by the ciliary body. Traditional external cyclodiode laser applied trans-sclerally is often reserved for eyes with end stage glaucoma and poor visual potential because of the risks of collateral damage, inflammation and hypotony. However endoscopic ablation of the ciliary body allows more targeted and titrated application of laser and is thought to be safer for this reason.

• Endoscopic Cyclophotocoagulation (ECP)

ECP applies a pulsed 810 nm diode laser to the ciliary body epithelium under direct visualisation via an endoscope and

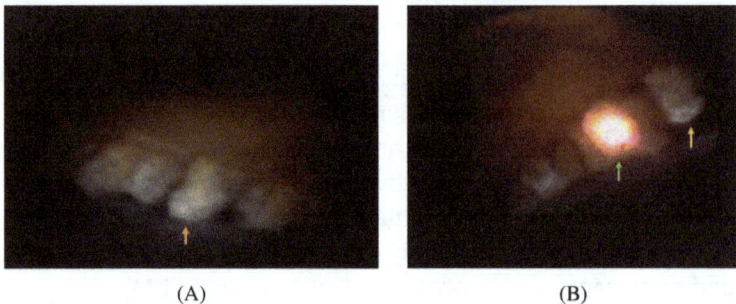

Fig. 7.10. ECP (A) Normal ciliary processes as seen through endoscope. (B) Treatment in progress. Seen are laser aiming beam (green arrow), and treated ciliary process which appears white (yellow arrow).

computer screen. The microprobe (Endo Optiks) is inserted via a clear corneal incision, usually at the end of phacoemulsification surgery, and laser is applied directly to the ciliary processes. The probe has a xenon light source as well as a helium neon laser aiming-beam to target the diode laser.

At least three quadrants (270°) are usually treated. The procedure can also be done as a standalone in pseudophakic eyes. With time the effect can wane as the ciliary body regenerates and re-perfuses, and therefore long-term outcomes may not be as promising as other procedures. Post-operative inflammation and cystoid macular oedema remain important considerations, and therefore ECP is not recommended in uveitic eyes or eyes prone to chronic inflammation. That said, several studies have reported good medium-term outcomes and shown effectiveness in IOP reduction and decreasing anti-glaucoma medication use.

ANGLE CLOSURE GLAUCOMAS

Lens Extraction

As the natural lens grows larger with age, it occupies a relatively larger volume. In a naturally smaller, hypermetropic eye this causes progressive angle closure and can on occasion precipitate acute angle closure attacks. Eyes with angle closure and raised IOP despite laser peripheral iridotomies may therefore require lens extraction surgery (phacoemulsification) if the lens is the main driver of angle closure. Ultrasound biomicroscopy (UBM) and anterior segment OCT are specialist imaging techniques that can help quantify the characteristics of eyes with angle closure and provide objective evidence of the need to remove the lens in order to open the drainage angles.

Goniosynechialysis

The MIGS procedures previously described are generally only possible if the anterior chamber drainage angle is open (i.e. in open-angle glaucomas). However if irido-trabecular adhesions (peripheral anterior synaechiae — PAS) exist due to angle closure, trabecular bypass or Schlemm Canal procedures are not possible due to inability to access the tissue. GSL is an ab

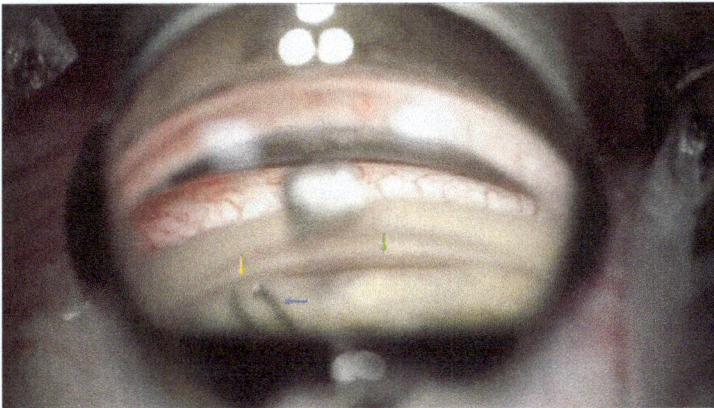

Fig. 7.11. Intra-operative view of goniosynechialysis. A 25-gauge forceps (blue arrow) is being used to gently pull the iris away from the angle structures in an area of angle closure (yellow arrow — trabecular meshwork barely visible). The green arrow indicates the area where the procedure has already been completed, with complete opening of the angle (ciliary body visualised).

interno technique that allows opening up of the angle structures by pulling away the peripheral iris tissue that has adhered to the TM, thereby re-establishing normal physiological outflow pathways. It is usually at the end of cataract surgery, via a clear corneal temporal incision and under direct gonioscopic visualisation, in small hypermetropic eyes with relatively large lenses. Cataract surgery alone will help reduce the pupil block mechanism in such eyes, but will not address any PAS formed.

8

IMPROVING QUALITY OF LIFE

Katie Smith and Pam Adams

GENERAL ADVICE AND MANAGEMENT

Maintaining and Improving Eyesight

An important role of an allied healthcare professional when dealing with a patient with glaucoma is to assess their visual acuity and visual fields and give practical advice, spectacles and low vision aids (where appropriate).

Another role is to check they are compliant with their medication (if prescribed). This will ensure they maintain and retain their visual fields and acuity. Their compliance in following prescribed treatment is key. It is surprising how many patients routinely stop taking their drops because 'they sting', they 'ran out' or they were just 'unsure what they were supposed to do'. Reinforcing the regime with a family member and contacting their GP will help with this. Difficulty instilling drops can be common with co-morbidities such as arthritis and clinicians should recommend instillation aids where appropriate. Patients also need to be informed that generally the drops will not cure their glaucoma; they just maintain their current level of sight. Again, many patients are under a misapprehension that the drops will give them back missing eyesight. This gentle management of a patient's expectations has benefits in years to come as the patient gains a better understanding of what is and what isn't possible.

Visual Acuity

Visual acuity measures can be variable in glaucoma. A patient may be unable to see the whole row of letters on a screen, or even locate the chart in the first place. Give them time and patience in assessing their acuity. It is important to realise that 6/6 vision can be a meaningless measure in patients where they have significant visual field (VF) loss. Assessment of their visual field has been discussed previously in this book but comparing the two VF plots (Fig. 8.1) shows what the variability can be, and how patient A would struggle significantly more than patient B — both having a diagnosis of POAG, and both being managed by ocular prostaglandins. Knowing that a patient has POAG (or any glaucoma diagnosis) is not enough to give them the best advice on managing their eyesight — it is imperative that the examiner knows what a patient's VF is too.

Accurate Refraction

An accurate refraction is a good starting point for improving a patient's life when they have glaucoma. When a patient is referred to secondary care from an optometrist or GP it is assumed that the hospital will take on their refractive care. Whilst this might be the case, it is not invariably so. Always check to see how old a person's spectacles are, and if over 1 year old then re-refract (It is important to use these results are used when selecting a lens for a visual field test to optimise results). LogMAR charts having the same number of letters on each line are a better way of assessing a patient's acuity rather than a standard Snellen chart (Fig. 8.2). It certainly makes the measure of VA in lower levels of acuity (6/24, LogMAR 0.6 and

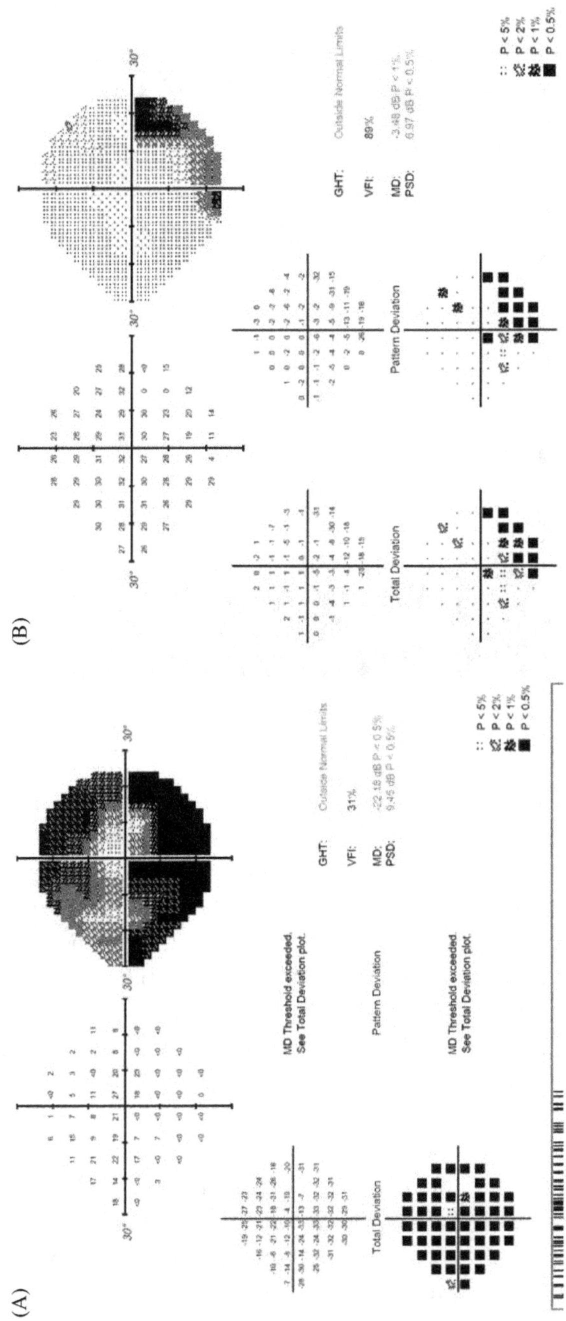
(A)
(B)
30°
Total Deviation
Pattern Deviation
MD Threshold exceeded.
See Total Deviation plot.
GHT:
Outside Normal Limits
VFI:
31%
MD:
-22.18 dB P < 0.5%
PSD:
9.46 dB P < 0.5%
89%
-3.98 dB P < 1%
6.97 dB P < 0.5%
P < 5%
P < 2%
P < 1%
P < 0.5%

Fig. 8.1.

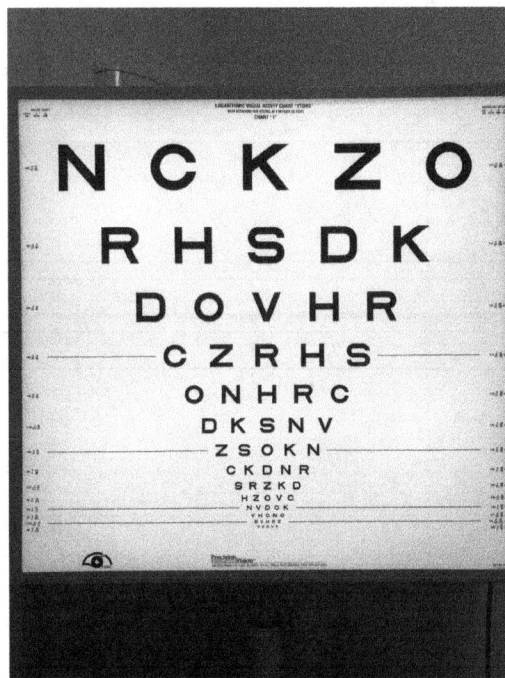

Fig. 8.2. LogMAR chart.

worse) much more accurate. A good rule of thumb is that when a change is detected, the patient should see at least one line of difference between their current prescription and a new pre-scription to get a 'noticeable' benefit. This is not a hard and fast rule, but saves the patient having unrealistic expectations of their new glasses. VF loss has an added complication of making many of the subjective tests (e.g. Jackson cross-cylinder, +1.00DS blur test) difficult and variable in nature. For example, as a patient is shown the two alternate lens positions in a cross-cylinder test, their fixation may move slightly and the target could fall into a scotoma thus being very difficult to see.

At this point the patient may be choosing where there is better fixation with a working part of their visual field, rather than the choice on cylinder axis and/or cylinder power. Where the cross-cylinder test is clearly hard to perform, a patient's astigmatism can be checked by less intensive means such as a fan and block test, or even directly from retinoscopy if the practitioner is confident of their retinoscopy skills.

Binocular Status

A common problem for glaucoma patients is maintaining single vision. Many will complain of diplopia whilst performing a distance task such as watching TV or driving. Others really struggle with reading and other near tasks. The reason for this, especially with advanced VF loss is that there is very little peripheral fusion lock: The subject's readily 'breakdown' to see two disparate images. Even if these images are joined with prism the lack of fusion means they readily decompensate to diplopic images when they move their eyes (e.g. when reading). A Fresnel prism is a quick means of assessing whether a patient can gain binocularity when they have diplopia, as it prevents them paying for spectacles that might not be successful. If the Fresnel does reduce or remove the diplopia it can be incorporated later on. If a patient can't be joined successfully with prisms it might be necessary to occlude one eye if the diplopia is troubling. When longstanding, a certain level of adaptation becomes evident and often the diplopia is rarely seen. In situations when the diplopia is intermittent it is worthwhile having a careful discussion with the patient to see which is going to be the best option; often it is a case of trial and error and working through the various options to find one that works.

MANAGING LOW VISION IN A GLAUCOMA PATIENT

Common Sense Advice for Glaucoma Patients with Visual Field Loss

As with other forms of vision loss, the three practical areas to advise a patient are illumination, contrast and magnification.

Using a good light is imperative for all concentrated near vision tasks. It is useful to demonstrate this improvement whilst the patient is in the testing chair, and this improvement may be several sizes of print. Ultimately the quality of the light source (its colour profile) is less important than its brightness. Relative Illumination (RI) is governed by the inverse square law (RI = $1/d^2$). For example, a light source at 1m is only 1/9 the brightness at 3 m, 1/16 the brightness at 4 m. Therefore, it is really important to keep the light source as close to the page as possible without it becoming a glare source — it should be level or slightly behind the observer to avoid this. The use of a good light applies to all tasks; thus a patient with glaucoma needs more light in the kitchen for cooking and eating and for any craft task (e.g. sewing, knitting).

Contrast sensitivity is commonly reduced with glaucoma, and whilst they can maintain good acuity in a test room where the letters are 100% contrast black on white, they can often struggle to read and see at home. Modern reading devices (electronic tablets and e-readers) have good contrast with illumination and this can be preferable to a traditional paper book or newspaper. For day to day problems like seeing the food on the plate contrast is very useful. A relatively dark meal such as stew is seen better off a white plate. A light-coloured meal, baked white fish for example, is easier to eat off a dark plate. A mug of tea is easier to pour when the tea is strong, and the mug is white. At home, stairs can be made more visible by applying contrasting carpet tape on the edge of the treads. Encourage patients to write using a bold black marker will make it easier for them to read back.

Mobility is a common problem for patients with glaucoma. With reduced VFs navigation is made much more difficult. Hazards such as an untidy floor, or head high open cupboard doors come into play. For patients with severe loss it is necessary to instruct the patient and their family to keep the floor clutter free, close all cupboard doors and, routinely either keep all doors at home closed or open to make entering and exiting a room less likely to end in a stumble, a trip or worse. Long cane mobility training, or the use of a guide dog is a possibility in severe visual field loss. Most hospital departments work with Eye Clinic Liaison Officers (ECLOs) who are there to give practical advice for daily living tasks, in association with Rehabilitation Officers for Visually Impaired (ROVIs — employed by local councils) who provide home visits and training to keep people mobile (such as long-cane technique).

Low Vision Aids for Glaucoma

Generally, with low vision, magnification is key. The most common cause of Sight Impairment (SI) registration is macular disease (dry or wet Age-related Macular Degeneration, Diabetic Macular Oedema, Retinal Vein Occlusion and hereditary retinal disorders). All these conditions lead to a central scotoma where the remaining eyesight (and potential) is governed by the retinal architecture (reduction in cone photoreceptor density away from the fovea), leading to the corresponding drop-off of VA with eccentric fixation. These patients respond well to enlargement of the retinal image as the object is magnified on to a working area of retina. As these conditions are more common with age, many patients with glaucoma may also have central retinal changes.

With glaucoma, the use of magnification is more subtle. If there is VF loss, yet still a working area close to fixation, magnification may make things worse. The enlarged words might then fall into a scotoma and become less visible. As mentioned earlier, it is well worth looking at the VF plot to see how close to fixation a working area is located. If it is close to fixation then the correct spectacle prescription and good light might be all that is needed. Low magnification can be obtained by increasing the near add towards 4.00 DS (1× magnification) and a corresponding focal length of 25 cm. For each doubling of magnification, the working distance (WD) halves (see Table 8.1 below). This close WD may also mean that if the patient is binocular at near, base-in prisms may need to be prescribed to achieve BSV and comfort.

At around 3× (12.00 DS addition) it becomes unfeasible to achieve the magnification with a high add. There are patients

Table 8.1. Effective magnification related to lens power and working distance.

	Lens power (DS)	Working distance
1×	+4.00	25 cm
2×	+8.00	12.5 cm
3×	+12.00	8.5 cm
4×	+16.00	6.7 cm
5×	+20.00	5 cm

Low Vision Appliances

+5.00 DS lens used as a simple magnifier

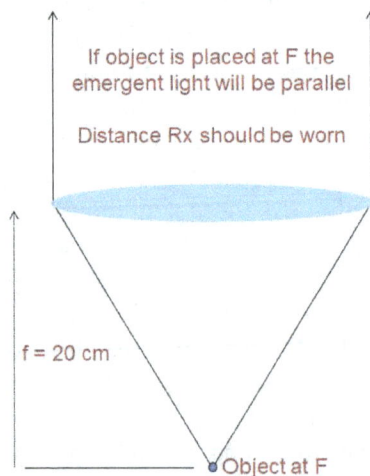

If object is placed at F the emergent light will be parallel

Distance Rx should be worn

f = 20 cm

Object at F

Fig. 8.3. (Courtesy of Andrew Keirl Opticians).

with specific needs who might be happy with this close WD (8.5 cm); most will not. For low power magnification 3× and above, to say 7×, hand-held magnifiers will suffice. On the higher strengths a stand-magnifier should be considered as it means the patient does not have to adjust the lens to achieve a focus. The lens is usually placed at the focal length of the lens meaning distance glasses are used to see the image, which is effectively seen at infinity (Fig. 8.3). Steady eye strategy, where the patient keeps their eyes still and the magnifier too but moves the page underneath is a really good idea. It helps to read this way as the patient is looking through the correct part of the magnifying lens, whereas if they move their eyes they may well be looking through a peripheral part of a high power lens with the attendant aberrations this will cause.

A simple and highly effective magnifier for glaucoma patients is a bright-field magnifier. This has three distinct advantages over conventional magnifiers. Firstly, light is concentrated from the surrounding room ambient light and is focused on the page. Secondly, it sits flat on the page and means there is no focusing necessary. Thirdly its low power magnification, typically 2–2.5× is an ideal magnification for patients with early to moderate VF loss (Fig. 8.4). As the patient moves it

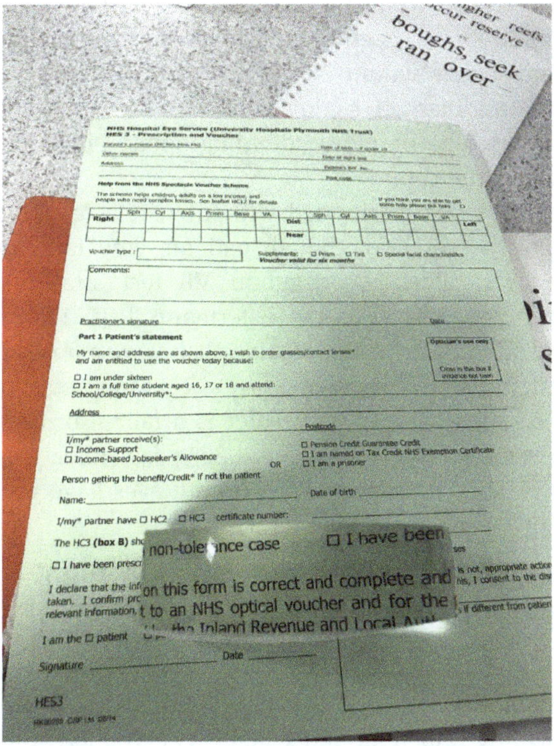

Fig. 8.4.

along the page it can help their proprioception, ensuring they read to the end of the line.

LEGAL IMPLICATIONS OF BEING DIAGNOSED WITH GLAUCOMA

Driving with Glaucoma

It is possible to drive with glaucoma (UK regulations) but the patient has to meet very strict VF guidelines in addition to the standard VA regulations (seeing a number plate at 20 m and able to read 6/12 corrected at least, monocular or binocular). Vision field requirements for safe driving are defined as 'a field of at least 120° on the horizontal measured using a target equivalent to the white Goldmann III4e settings. In addition, there should be no significant defect in the binocular field which encroaches within 20° of fixation above or below the horizontal meridian'. A significant defect has been defined by the DVLA as four or more adjoining spots, either wholly or partly within the central 20°.

This test is best performed without spectacles (in case the frame gives a scotoma), though patients who fail can ask to re-sit the test aided. A common VF test strategy on the Humphrey VF analyser is the Estermann Test. 120 spots are presented supra-threshold and false positive responses (no light presented but the patient presses) are monitored. Any false positive response of 20% or greater is a fail — or of course if they don't have 120° VF, or central 20° pass either. It is a legal duty for patients to inform DVLA if both eyes have glaucoma.

Registration (Sight Impaired, Severely Sight Impaired) with Glaucoma

Registration as SI or SSI is possible with glaucoma, even if the VA is technically too good to meet the criterion. When the VF is significantly impaired, and when it is extremely impaired SI and SSI registration can be considered.

Generally, to be certified as **severely sight impaired (blind)**, your sight must fall into one of the following categories, while wearing any glasses or contact lenses that you may need:

• Visual acuity of less than 3/60 with a full visual field.
• Visual acuity between 3/60 and 6/60 with a severe reduction of field of vision, such as tunnel vision.
• Visual acuity of 6/60 or above but with an extremely reduced field of vision, especially if a lot of sight is missing in the lower part of the field.

To be certified as **sight impaired (partially sighted)** your sight must fall into one of the following categories, while wearing any glasses or contact lenses that you may need:

• Visual acuity of 3/60 to 6/60 with a full field of vision.
• Visual acuity of up to 6/24 with a moderate reduction of field of vision or with a central part of vision that is cloudy or blurry.
• Visual acuity of 6/18 or even better if a large part of your field of vision, for example, a whole half of your vision, is missing or a lot of your peripheral vision is missing.

9

DEVELOPING A HOLISTIC APPROACH TO GLAUCOMA MANAGEMENT

Michael Smith

When caring for glaucoma patients, it is important to remember that the ultimate aim of glaucoma treatment is to prevent visual disability. When discussing glaucoma treatment we almost always talk about Intraocular Pressure (IOP). This is logical because many studies have shown that IOP reduction is directly linked to preservation of the visual field and therefore maintenance of good functional vision. However, from both research studies and our experience of glaucoma practice we know that there is great variability in the relationships between IOP and visual field loss, and between visual field loss and day-to-day visual problems. In addition, even a simple change in treatment can have significant downsides, both in terms of side effects and inconvenience, but again this can vary between individual patients. It is therefore important to consider the individual patient when making treatment decisions. Below is a discussion of the factors the glaucoma clinician should consider when advising glaucoma patients on their treatment options.

DOES THE IOP NEED TO BE LOWER?

In a minority of glaucoma cases the IOP is very high (e.g. >30 mhg, or significantly lower if glaucoma more severe) and carries a high risk of visual loss in the short to medium term. In this situation treatment should be started or, if already on treatment, increased to reduce the IOP and preserve the vision. In the majority of cases however, the risk to vision is a long term one and before increasing treatment the clinician should consider the points below.

WHAT EVIDENCE IS THERE OF GLAUCOMA PROGRESSION?

In patients on long term glaucoma treatment it is not uncommon for the IOP to increase over time, or for the visual field or optic disc to show evidence of progression. Before automatically increasing treatment the clinician should look for evidence of progression. If there is an IOP rise and no evidence of progression, then consideration should be given to accepting the rise in IOP and continuing to monitor. Whether this is the correct decision for the individual patient depends on several factors, including the history of the individual patient in terms of IOP and progression, but the factors discussed below should also be considered.

IS THE PROGRESSION LIKELY TO THREATEN FUNCTIONAL VISION?

Studies have shown that the majority of glaucoma patients progress over time. The aim of treatment is not to prevent *any* progression but rather to ensure that this progression does not result in visual disability during the patient's lifespan. Just because the optic disc or visual field is showing evidence that the glaucoma is worsening does not mean treatment automatically needs to be increased, particularly if the progression is slow and the treatment carries a significant risk of side effects or inconvenience to the patient. Again, this requires assessment of the individual patient's clinical and personal situation but is particularly relevant in the elderly population where life expectancy may be limited, and the impact of increasing treatment can be considerable.

IS THE PATIENT USING THEIR CURRENT TREATMENT?

Before increasing treatment, it is important to ensure the patient is using their current treatment correctly. We do know that the rate of adherence to glaucoma treatment is often poor, and this is more likely in patients with memory problems or difficulties instilling the drops. Increasing treatment in this situation may make adherence worse, and our efforts are likely to be better concentrated on helping patient overcome the barriers to good adherence to their current treatment.

WHAT IS THE RISK OF INCREASING TREATMENT?

This question covers several aspects of the downsides of treatment. If surgery is being considered, we should always ensure the risk of visual loss from surgery is not higher than the risk of visual loss from glaucomatous progression. Will an increase in drop treatment in a patient with ocular surface symptoms make this worse? The inconvenience of an increase in treatment should also be considered. For example, in a patient using prostaglandin/beta-blocker drops once daily if we wish to increase treatment, we would commonly add a carbonic anhydrase inhibitor drop twice daily. Although this may seem an easy thing to do in clinic, to the patient this represents a threefold increase in treatment. This is a significant increase for anyone, but for those who already take many other medicines or who rely on others to instil their drops this could have a big impact on their quality of life. We need to be certain the increased treatment is necessary.

HOW PRACTICAL IS AN INCREASE IN TREATMENT?

Although we do often consider side effects when making treatment decisions, we are not so good at considering the wider impact this may have on a patient's life. Could the patient who lives many miles from hospital come for the 6 or more visits to outpatients needed after trabeculectomy? Could the daughter of the elderly patient who struggles to visit her every day to instil her drops cope if the drops were increased to twice daily? How about the wife of the glaucoma patient with dementia who resists the drops on most days? We won't know unless we ask.

WHAT DOES THE PATIENT THINK?

Shared decision making is defined as the conversation that happens between a patient and their health professional to reach a healthcare choice together. It is a move away from the traditional paternalistic doctor-patient relationship and towards a "no decision about me, without me" model of care. We do know that patients who are actively involved in decisions about their care are more likely to engage with treatment. As we've discussed glaucoma management involves balancing the benefits of treatment against the side effects and inconvenience of this treatment. In an individual patient the exact position of this balance is affected by the individual patient's attitude to risk. Some patients will prefer significant side effects and inconvenience to even a small chance of visual loss, whereas others will only accept medical intervention if the risk of visual loss is high. Again, we won't know unless we ask.

ROLE OF CLINICAL GUIDELINES

There are a variety of guidelines on glaucoma management. Clinician guidelines are intended to serve as an indicator of what is considered best practice for the majority of patients the majority of the time. This does not mean they must be followed to the line in every single case and clinicians have a responsibility to consider what is best for the individual patient, taking into account the factors discussed above. When deviating from clinical guidelines it is important for the clinician to document the reasons for this clearly in the clinical records.

ROLE OF THE GLAUCOMA PRACTITIONER

Most glaucoma care in the UK is multidisciplinary and all members of the team have a role in ensuring the correct decision is made for each individual patient. For example, although the consultant may be best placed to discuss with the patient the ins and outs of glaucoma surgery, the input of other members of the team with respect to the patient's views and the impact of any treatment escalation on the patient are as important in the final decision on whether to proceed with surgery. Practitioners, in particular, can play an important role in the decision-making process, as they often spend more time with individual patients than the consultant and may appear more approachable.

USEFUL RESOURCES

Royal College of Ophthalmologists — www.rcophth.ac.uk
American Academy of Ophthalmology — www.aao.org
International Glaucoma Association — www.glaucoma-association.com
Royal National Institute of Blind People — www.rnib.org.uk
National Institute for Health and Care Excellence — www.nice.org.uk
World Glaucoma Association — www.wga.one
European Glaucoma Society — www.eugs.org
Atlas of Gonioscopy — www.gonioscopy.org
Iowa Glaucoma Curriculum — www.curriculum.iowaglaucoma.org

USEFUL RESOURCES

Royal College of Ophthalmologists — www.rcophth.ac.uk
American Academy of Ophthalmology — www.aao.org
International Glaucoma Association — www.glaucoma-association.com
Royal National Institute of Blind People — www.rnib.org.uk
National Institute for Health and Care Excellence — www.nice.org.uk
World Glaucoma Association — www.wga.one
European Glaucoma Society — www.eugs.org
Atlas of Gonioscopy — www.gonioscopy.org
Iowa Glaucoma Curriculum — www.curriculum.iowaglaucoma.org

INDEX

www.ingramcontent.com/pod-product-compliance
Lightning Source LLC
LaVergne TN
LVHW010748070225

803128LV00004B/546